Laparoscopic Sacrocolpopexy for Beginners

Peter von Theobald

Laparoscopic Sacrocolpopexy for Beginners

How to Start if you Never Dared Before?

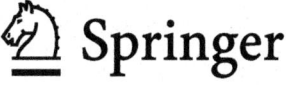 Springer

Peter von Theobald
Service de Gynécologie et Obstétrique
Centre d'Études Périnatales de l'Océan Indien (CEPOI) - EA7388
CHU Réunion, Hôpital Félix Guyon
Saint Denis de la Réunion
France

Additional material to this book can be downloaded from http://extras.springer.com.

ISBN 978-3-319-57635-0   ISBN 978-3-319-57636-7   (eBook)
DOI 10.1007/978-3-319-57636-7

Library of Congress Control Number: 2017941724

Printed on acid-free paper

This Springer imprint is published by Springer Nature
The registered company is Springer International Publishing AG
The registered company address is: Gewerbestrasse 11, 6330 Cham, Switzerland

Foreword

This foreword is aiming to explain why I decided to write this book.

I started as resident in Gynecology and Obstetrics in 1983 at the university hospital of Caen, Normandy, France and became consultant at the same place in 1987. I stayed at the university hospital because of my passion for teaching and for developing new techniques and new technology. In Caen, we had a pioneer team for laparoscopic surgery, including gynecologists and bowel surgeons. We organized starting from 1988 a huge lot of post graduate trainings, master class sessions, on hands training almost every week, and a big congress in Deauville every year. We were also pioneers for vaginal surgery, without mesh until 1998 (but very few people came to train because laparoscopy was more trendy), and with vaginal mesh afterwards (many people came, let's guess why). Thus, I also had the chance to be invited in so many places all over the world to give talks and perform live operations and I could meet a lot of wonderful, inventive and over skilled people that helped me to improve daily. I must admit that LSCP has always been my favorite operation.

I realized after all those years of teaching that LSCP was perceived by many surgeons as a very difficult and dangerous technique and most of them, even if they had come to my OR for hands on training, if they had watched tenth of live LSCP in many congresses and seen a lot of videos, most of them didn't dare to schedule their own first procedure. That means that it isn't enough to teach, to show, to perform. You need to write it down in a very pragmatic and pedagogic way to complete the practical training.

That's why I've decided to write this book, fruit of my 30 years experience in the field of gynecologic and urogynecologic surgery, having personally performed more than 600 LSCP since 1993. I wanted to help the young surgeon to progress before the first procedure to reach the level of skill, to explain how to choose the first patient, to help him during the operation that is described step by step with pictures and drawings, also if things go wrong with tips for troubleshooting. I wanted to show tricks to spare time, to make some steps of the LSCP easier to perform. Alternative techniques, concomitant hysterectomy or not, stress incontinence repair at the same time or not, long term results, post operative care, every chapter in my book is based on practical experience and aiming to give a synthetic answer to the question a beginner in LSCP might ask.

LSCP is one of the essential procedures to treat Pelvic Organ Prolapse (POP). It is not the only one; vaginal surgery is as indispensable. There are specific indications for each approach. These indications are largely discussed in this book. A modern urogynecologist should master all of them and choose the correct technique for the right patient. I deeply hope that this book, the first "cookbook" about LSCP for beginners ever written, will be a big help for the young surgeons who are longing to perform this beautiful operation.

Contents

Pelvic organ prolapse (POP) has been described as a major female health issue for all of time. Around 1550 B.C.E., the Ebers papyrus recommended to rub the body of the patient with petroleum or with manure and honey to put the womb back in place. Hippocrates (460–377 B.C.E.) thought that the uterus acted as an animal unto itself. He recommended fumigations to stimulate the uterus to retreat.

Correct anatomical knowledge occurred much later, thanks to illegal cadaver dissections starting in the sixteenth century. Andreus Vesalius, professor of anatomy at Padua, with his book "De Corporis Humani Fabrica" stated an accurate description of the entire female genital tract including the ligaments of the uterus and helped to better understand female pelvic floor anatomy. Alwin Mackenrodt published his description of the female pelvic floor connective tissue in 1895 and Bonney published "The Principles that Should Underlie All Operations for Prolapse" in 1934. Their work would later inspire DeLancey in 1992 to describe the levels of fascial support and Petros for his integral theory in 2001 [1].

Evolution of surgery was mainly related to anatomical knowledge and the beginning of anesthesiology. The first vaginal hysterectomy for uterine prolapse was reported by Choppin, of New Orleans, in 1861. In 1892, Zweifel of Germany, in his book, commented on his attempts to correct uterovaginal prolapse by using silkworm sutures to fix the upper vagina to the sacrotuberous ligament. In 1937 vaginal hysterectomy had become the predominant operation, but quickly, vault prolapse became a recognized complication. In 1927, Miller described the bilateral, transperitoneal iliococcygeus suspension for vault prolapse. In 1957, McCall, published his technique of obliterating the cul-de-sac of Douglas to cure an enterocele and prevent vault prolapse.

The birth of sacrocolpopexy (SCP) and sacrocolpohysteropexy (SCHP): in 1957, Arthure and Savage from London recognized that vault prolapse could occur after abdominal or vaginal hysterectomy and that hysterectomy alone would not

Downing KT. Uterine Prolapse: From Antiquity to Today. Obstet Gynecol Int. 2012;2012:649459. doi:10.1155/2012/649459.

© Springer International Publishing AG 2017
P. von Theobald, *Laparoscopic Sacrocolpopexy for Beginners*,
DOI 10.1007/978-3-319-57636-7_1

cure uterine prolapse. They published their "Uterine prolapse and prolapse of the vaginal vault treated by sacral hysteropexy" the same year as Ameline and Huguier from Paris published "Posterior suspension to the lumbo-sacral disk; abdominal method of replacement of the utero-sacral ligament" [2]. One year later, in 1958, Huguier and Scali published the first series of results: "Posterior suspension of the genital axis on the lumbosacral disk in the treatment of uterine prolapse" [3]. These three publications describe the technique that has remained almost identical to the abdominal technique performed today.

Laparoscopic sacrocolpopexy (LSCP) and sacrocolpohysteropexy (LSCHP) started in 2000–2001 with four publications [4–7] describing the technique and the first results of that procedure performed since the early nineties by these French teams: Michel Cosson in Lille, Arnaud Wattiez in Clermont Ferrand, Angelique Cheret and Peter von Theobald in Caen.

In our team, in Caen, first LSCHP was performed in 1993. At that time, alternative techniques to abdominal SCP were only vaginal procedures, mainly sacrospinous ligament suspensions, myorraphies and colporraphies of various kinds. The only vaginal uterus preserving technique was the ancient (1908) Manchester-Fothergill procedure frequently associated to cervix amputation (1915). What motivated us to start LSCP and LSCHP was the combination of a minimal invasive approach with tissue reinforcement by synthetic mesh. Thus, we were expecting better results, less post operative pain and earlier discharge from the hospital.

References

1. Petros PP, Skilling PM. Pelvic floor rehabilitation in the female according to the integral theory of female urinary incontinence. First report. Eur J Obstet Gynecol Reprod Biol. 2001 Feb;94(2):264–9.
2. Ameline A, Huguier J. Posterior suspension to the lumbo-sacral disk; abdominal method of replacement of the utero-sacral ligaments. Gynecol Obstet (Paris). 1957 Jan–Mar;56(1):94–8.
3. Huguier J, Scali P. Posterior suspension of the genital axis on the lumbosacral disk in the treatment of uterine prolapse. Presse Med. 1958 May 3;66(35):781–4.
4. Cosson M, Bogaert E, Narducci F, Querleu D. Crépin G Laparoscopic sacral colpopexy: short-term results and complications in 83 patients. J Gynecol Obstet Biol Reprod (Paris). 2000 Dec;29(8):746–50.
5. Wattiez A, Canis M, Mage G, Pouly JL, Bruhat MA. Promontofixation for the treatment of prolapse. Urol Clin North Am. 2001 Feb;28(1):151–7.
6. Cheret A, Von Theobald P, Lucas J, Dreyfus M, Herlicoviez M. Laparoscopic promontofixation feasibility study in 44 patients. J Gynecol Obstet Biol Reprod (Paris). 2001 Apr;30(2):139–43.
7. von Theobald P. Laparoscopic promontofixation. J Chir (Paris). 2001 Dec;138(6):353–7.

Physiopathology of POP

Etiology of POP is multifactorial. Most of them are well known. Pelvic floor traumatisms as provoked by pregnancy and vaginal delivery are very important. They are responsible for tissue elongation, nerve and vessel damage, elastic tissue breaks. Postmenopausal atrophy of the pelvic floor tissues is another well-demonstrated factor, frequently destabilizing a pre-existing injury. Obesity and chronic bronchial obstructive disease increase the risk of prolapse.

One of the main risk factors for POP is the quality of the connective tissue in the pelvis and the perineum. Many series are now available, assessing samples of uterosacral ligaments, vaginal tissue from the apex, from the anterior wall, from the Paraurethral position. Significant modifications are pointed out. For the apex, smooth muscle cells and collagen III as well as active matrix metalloproteinase 9 (MMP 9) concentrations are raised in POP [1, 2]. For the uterosacral ligaments, collagen density, collagen III and Tenascin concentrations are raised in POP with a decrease in Elastin [3–5]. Only one series [6] finds no significant difference in uterosacral ligaments as in vaginal tissue. But the exact site of vaginal tissue sampling is not described in the paper. There are different variations in apex tissue and uterosacral ligaments compared to anterior vaginal wall or paraurethral tissue, where collagen III, I and VI concentrations, Vitronectin expression and extra cellular matrix density are reduced in POP [7–10]. Another publication reveals reduced amount of smooth muscle cells in the round ligaments of patients with POP [11]. All authors insist on the alterations of the extra cellular matrix of the pelvic floor connective tissue associated with decrease of smooth muscle cells. The tissue of the fascias and the ligaments is less elastic and more breakable.

The real question is: are these changes aetiology or consequence of the POP? Three publications tend to underline the primary weakness of the collagen in POP. A recent study [12] has shown positive correlation between low bone densitometry and pelvic organ prolapse (POP). As we know that osteoporosis is first a disease of the collagen matrix of the bone, especially of its turnover, we can imagine a similar mechanism for POP. Furthermore, a review upon SERM in 2006 [13] shows very diverse effects of SERM on POP: Some, like Raloxifen, are protective while some

© Springer International Publishing AG 2017
P. von Theobald, *Laparoscopic Sacrocolpopexy for Beginners*,
DOI 10.1007/978-3-319-57636-7_2

others have been retrieved from trials because of their POP inducing effects. Knowing that SERM are modifying the expression of several genes involved in collagen turnover and extra cellular matrix integrity, we can argue that a dysfunction of these genes leads to connective tissue breakdown and POP. Another paper has established a strong association (OR3.12, $p < 0.05$) between two connective tissue disorders: striae and POP [14].

It appears that genetically induced bad connective tissue or premature ageing of this tissue may be the "primum movens" of POP. But we all know that small prolapses are likely to regress in time. Handa in 2004 has confirmed these data [15]: regression rate for grade 1 prolapses after 2–8 years is 23.5% for cystocoele, 22% for rectocele and 48% for uterine prolapse. Progression rates are only 9.5%, 13.5% and 1.9% respectively. This means that many women undergo vaginal distension and distortion at the time of the delivery, but most of them are able to repair properly their tissues. Furthermore, undergoing the same mechanical stress, different patients may have various degrees of pelvic floor tissue injuries. The degree is correlated to the elasticity and the resistance of their connective tissue.

To summarize, we can say that POP is due to distension and/or disruption of weak, fibrous and inelastic connective tissue possibly associated to decreased ability to repair it. Thus, a correct repair should fix the anatomic disruptions or distensions and improve the quality of the supportive tissue.

References

1. Badiou W, Granier G, Bousquet PJ, et al. Comparative histological analysis of anterior vaginal wall in women with pelvic organ prolapse or control subjects. Int Urogynecol J Pelvic Floor Dysfunct. 2008;19(5):723–9.
2. Moalli PA, Shand SH, Zyczynski HM, et al. Remodeling of vaginal connective tissue in patients with prolapse. Obstet Gynecol. 2005;106(5 Pt 1):953–63.
3. Goepel C. Differential elastin and tenascin immunolabeling in the uterosacral ligaments in postmenopausal women with and without pelvic organ prolapse. Acta Histochem. 2008;110(3):204–9.
4. Suzme R, Yalcin O, Gurdol F, et al. Connective tissue alterations in women with pelvic organ prolapse and urinary incontinence. Acta Obstet Gynecol Scand. 2007;86(7):882–8.
5. Gabriel B, Denschlag D, Göbel H, et al. Uterosacral ligament in postmenopausal women with or without pelvic organ prolapse. Int Urogynecol J Pelvic Floor Dysfunct. 2005;16(6):475–9.
6. Phillips CH, Anthony F, Benyon C, Monga AK. Collagen metabolism in the uterosacral ligaments and vaginal skin of women with uterine prolapse. BJOG. 2006;113(1):39–46.
7. Song Y, Hong X, Yu Y, Lin Y. Changes of collagen type III and decorin in paraurethral connective tissue from women with stress urinary incontinence and prolapse. Int Urogynecol J Pelvic Floor Dysfunct. 2007;18(12):1459–63.
8. Lin SY, Tee YT, Ng SC, et al. Changes in the extracellular matrix in the anterior vagina of women with or without prolapse. Int Urogynecol J Pelvic Floor Dysfunct. 2007;18(1):43–8.
9. Goepel C, Hefler L, Methfessel HD, Koelbl H. Periurethral connective tissue status of postmenopausal women with genital prolapse with and without stress incontinence. Acta Obstet Gynecol Scand. 2003;82(7):659–64.
10. Söderberg MW, Falconer C, Byström B, et al. Young women with genital prolapse have a low collagen concentration. Acta Obstet Gynecol Scand. 2004;83(12):1193–8.

11. Ozdegirmenci O, Karslioglu Y, Dede S, et al. Smooth muscle fraction of the round ligament in women with pelvic organ prolapse: a computer-based morphometric analysis. Int Urogynecol J Pelvic Floor Dysfunct. 2005;16(1):39–43; discussion 43.

12. Pal L, Hailpern SM, Santoro NF, et al. Association of pelvic organ prolapse and fractures in postmenopausal women: analysis of baseline data from the Women's Health Initiative estrogen plus progestin trial. Menopause. 2008;15(1):59–66.

13. Cox DA, Helvering LM. Extracellular matrix integrity: a possible mechanism for differential clinical effects among selective estrogen receptor modulators and estrogens? Mol Cell Endocrinol. 2006;247(1–2):53–9.

14. Salter SA, Batra RS, Rohrer TE, et al. Striae and pelvic relaxation: two disorders of connective tissue with a strong association. J Invest Dermatol. 2006;126(8):1745–8.

15. Handa VL, Garrett E, Hendrix S, et al. Progression and remission of pelvic organ prolapse: a longitudinal study of menopausal women. Am J Obstet Gynecol. 2004;190(1):27–32.

Anatomy

3.1   Fascias, Ligaments, Organs and Levels Simplified

My aim is neither to go into sophisticated description of detailed functional anatomy nor to explain again the integral theory according to P.P. Petros [1]. I just want to stress out the main structures responsible for pelvic static in order to explain how LSCP can help to repair POP.

On Fig. 3.1, you see the pelvic fascia underlined by the elevator muscles. The pelvic fascia is a hammock stretched out between the pubis and the sacrum at the top of the elevator muscles. The anterior part is fragile because three orifices cross the hammock; one for the urethra, one for the vagina and one for the anal canal. Most POPs occur through the main defect, the vaginal slot.

The posterior part of the fascia is very resistant because nothing opens it and the elevator plate underneath is very resistant.

Laterally, you notice the arcus tendineus fascia pelvis.

On Fig. 3.2, you see how the rectum is positioned. The anal canal goes through the hammock whilst the proximal part of the rectum is lying on the resistant part of the structure, the elevator plate. An increase of intra-abdominal pressure coming from above (arrow) will push the rectum against the elevator plate instead of pressing it through one of the orifices. The rectum can be maintained above the elevator plate by small forces due to fascia adhesion.

On Fig. 3.3, you see the shape of the vagina, starting as a vertical slot at the vulva, crossing the elevator muscles and the pelvic fascia, kinking just above and lying on the rectum and the pelvic fascia, becoming a horizontal flat structure attached laterally to the fascia and to the arcus tendineus fascia pelvis. Here again, a pressure coming from above will press the vagina as the rectum on the elevator plate as long as there are some anchoring structures, securing the vagina to this position.

Figure 3.4 shows similar positioning of the bladder above the elevator plate. But, unfortunately, due to its anterior position, a large part of the posterior wall of the

© Springer International Publishing AG 2017
P. von Theobald, *Laparoscopic Sacrocolpopexy for Beginners*,
DOI 10.1007/978-3-319-57636-7_3

Fig. 3.1 The bare pelvic
fascia

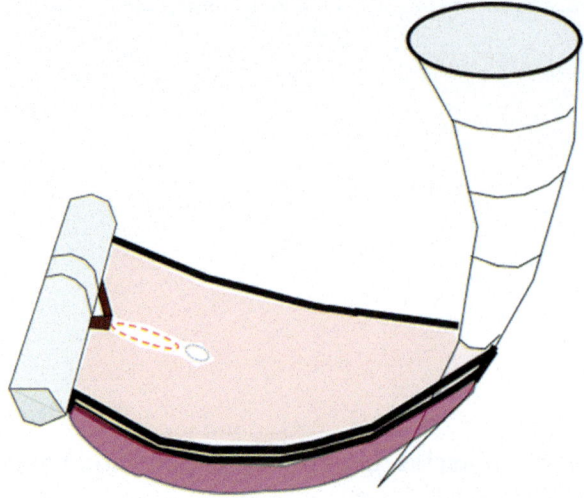

Fig. 3.2 The rectum and
the pelvic fascia

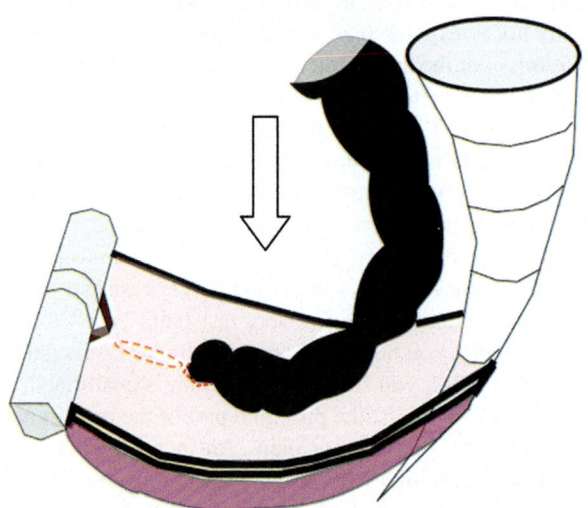

bladder stays just above the fragile part of the hammock, above the vaginal slot. This explains easily why the bladder is so frequently involved in POP. Lateral attachment of the bladder to the arcus tendineus fascia pelvis is usually strong as is its fixation to the cervix (both in blue lines).

You notice that the cervix is surrounded by many attachments: to the vesicovaginal fascia anteriorly, laterally to the Cardinal ligaments and posteriorly to the rectovaginal fascia and to the uterosacral ligaments. This constitutes the pericervical ring which acts like a keystone to the pelvic floor.

Fig. 3.3 Rectum, vagina and the pelvic fascia

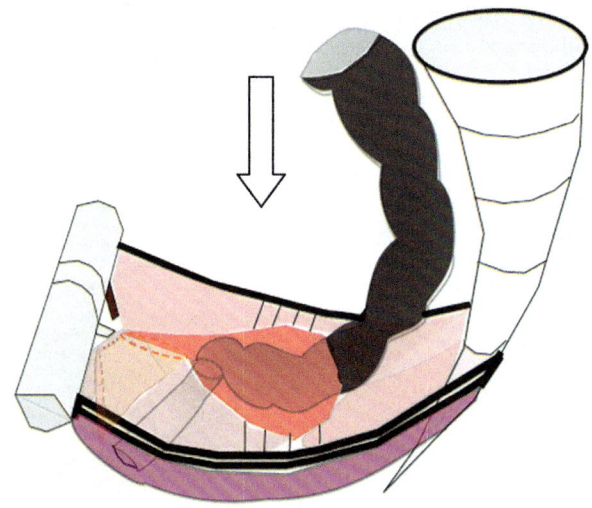

Fig. 3.4 Bladder, uterine cervix, vagina and rectum on the pelvic fascia

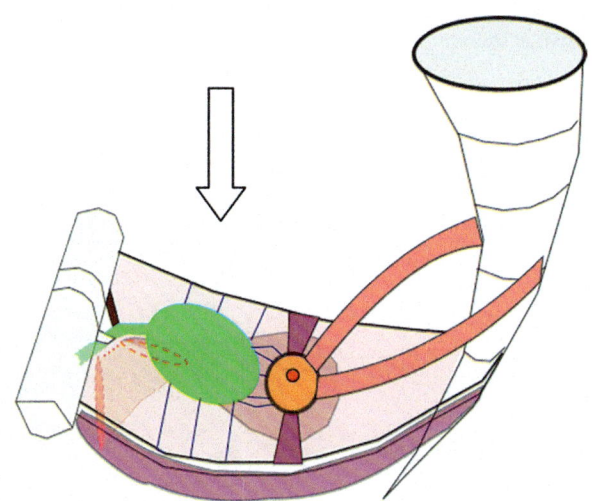

Figure 3.5 shows how the structures articulate to each other.

Figure 3.6 shows how it changes at stress, the anteverted uterine body is pushed anteriorly towards the pubis bone, the uterine cervix is pushed backwards with the vaginal cul de sac and the rectum and thus, the vesicovaginal fascia is stretched in order to avoid cystocele. The rectovaginal fascia is stretched as well. This is to demonstrate the usefulness of the uterus to prevent POP and to explain why vaginal vault prolapse is so frequent.

Fig. 3.5 The complete
pelvis at rest

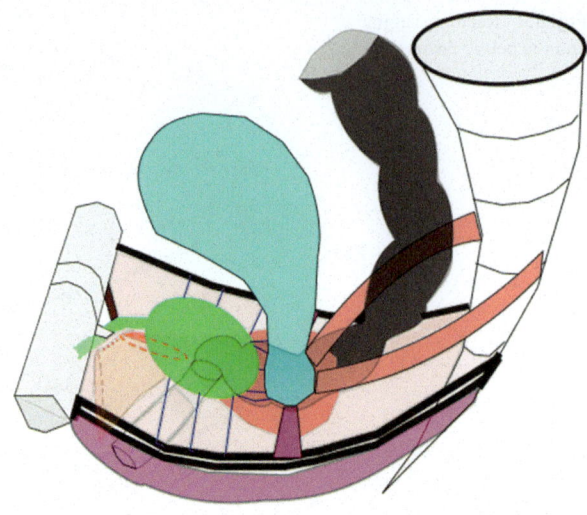

Fig. 3.6 The complete
pelvis at stress

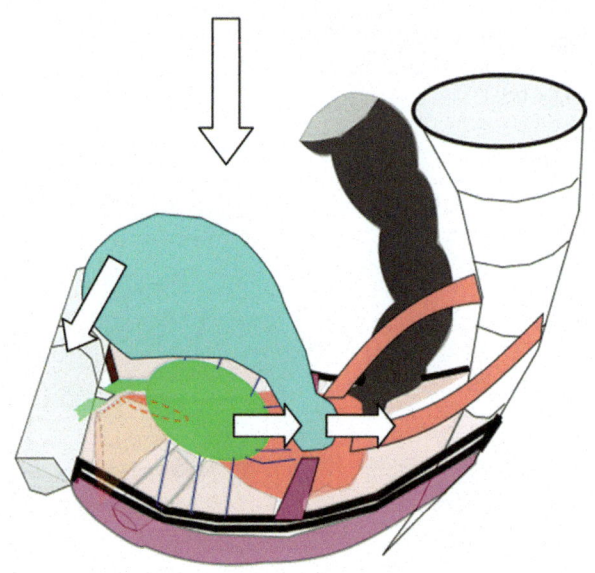

Figure 3.7 shows the three levels of fixation of the pelvic organs: level 1 is every structure securing the cervix and the vaginal posterior cul de sac. It includes mainly the uterosacral ligaments, the lateral Cardinal ligaments and the fascial adhesions to the elevator plate. Level 2 fixation id relaying on the vesicovaginal and the recto-vaginal fascias and on their insertions to the lateral attachments (arcus tendineus fascia pelvis) and to the pericervical ring. Level 3 is holding the distal part of the pelvic organs, below the pelvic fascia. Adhesion or fusion of the three organs among a dense muscular and fibrous structure (perineal body in grey) constitutes the perineum.

Fig. 3.7 The levels

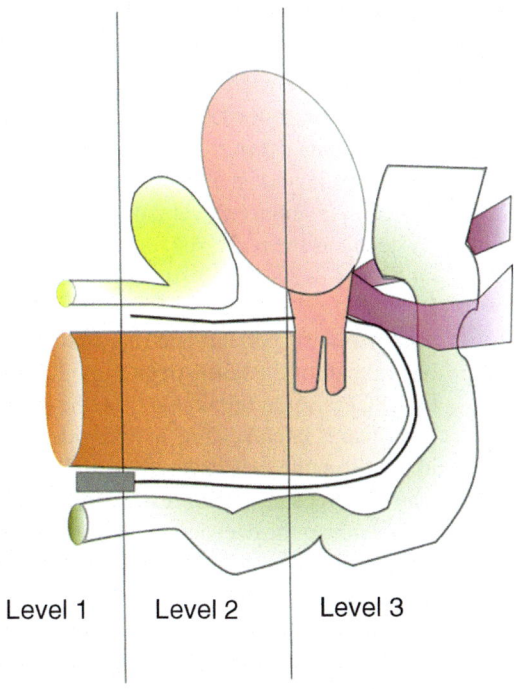

Level 1 | Level 2 | Level 3

3.2 The Lesions

1. Lesions of level 1: Level 1 lesions are easy to identify because they are due to rupture, desinsertion or elongation of the cardinal and uterosacral ligaments. The uterus or the vaginal vault slides away from the levator plate, pulling the Douglas pouch with him, invaginating the vagina and descending more or less though the space between the levator muscles. Hysterocele (uterine descent) or trachelocele (descent of the uterine cervix), vault prolapse (after hysterectomy), enterocele (very frequently associated) is diagnosed clinically with a speculum by pulling on the cervix or the vault with a Kugel forceps. Cervical elongation should be evaluated at this stage because this lesion will not be repaired by LSCP, needing a shortening through vaginal approach. Enterocele is a posterior colpocele starting at the upper part of the posterior vaginal wall. It may be mixed up with rectocele, and frequently a rectal toucher is necessary to differentiate.
2. Level 2 lesions are of two kinds: rectocele (a posterior colpocele) and cystocele (an anterior colpocele). Very detailed examination is crucial at level 2 because some of these lesions are likely to be cured by LSCP and others not.
   (a) Concerning posterior level 2 defects:
   The rectovaginal fascia, also called Denonvilliers aponevrosis, is spread between the anterior rectal wall and the posterior vaginal wall, anchored laterally to the pelvic wall, to the pericervical ring at the top and to the levator muscles at the bottom. Lesions, frequently tears due to obstetrical history, may be central or

lateral, high or low, unique or multiple. Lateral defects may frequently be associated to defects in the levator muscles as shown by MRI studies.

Repair of all posterior defects is possible with LSCP. It is even a specially good indication for LSCP because, if you are opening the rectovaginal dissection plane down to the elevators, you may reinforce with the mesh, the whole fascia and its attachments.

(b) Concerning anterior level 2 defects:

Cystocele is the real issue for LSCP. Anterior level 2 defects are summarized on Figs. 3.8, 3.9, and 3.10.

Lesions may occur in the vesico vaginal fascia at the upper part, tearing it away from the pericervical ring (a on Figs. 3.8 and 3.9) or be located at the central part of the fascia (c on Figs. 3.8 and 3.9). These lesions may be cured by LSCP; as you see on Fig. 3.8, the mesh will cover these defects.

If the tear is lateral on one or both sides (b on Fig. 3.8), as there is no possibility to attach the mesh laterally with LSCP, the defect will remain and no cure may be expected. Thus, it is crucial to diagnose the type of anterior defect before taking the decision to proceed to LSCP. Clinical examination may find the anterior colpocele very smooth, flat and thin with deep lateral cul de sacs and a central or upper defect is likely. If the vaginal prolapsed mucosa is remaining thick and wrinkled with no more lateral cul de sac, a lateral defect should be suspected and a vaginal procedure discussed. Photo 1 shows a typical central defect and Photo 2 a lateral defect. Be aware that defects can be multiple and combined and then, correct diagnosis may be difficult.

Last possible type of defect is an accompanying cystocele: the uterus stays attached to an intact vesicovaginal fascia and the uterine descent pulls down this fascia and the attached bladder (Fig. 3.10). Clinically, the vaginal mucosa is thick and wrinkled and the cystocele is completely reduced when you push back in place the uterus. In fact, it is only a level 1 defect.

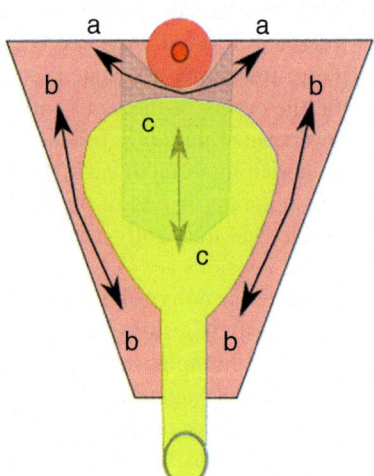

Fig. 3.8 Vesico vaginal fascia and its possible defects: rupture from the cervix (**a**), lateral defect (**b**), medial defect (**c**). The anterior mesh is in place

Fig. 3.9 Profile showing medial defect of the vesico vaginal fascia (**c**) and rupture from the cervix (**a**)

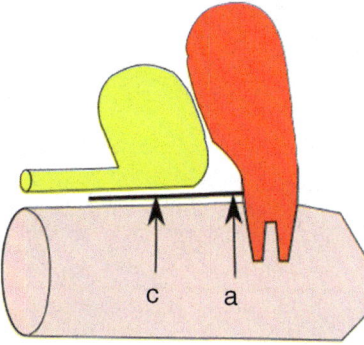

Fig. 3.10 Cystocele accompanying an uterine prolapse (hysterocele) without defect in the vesicovaginal fascia

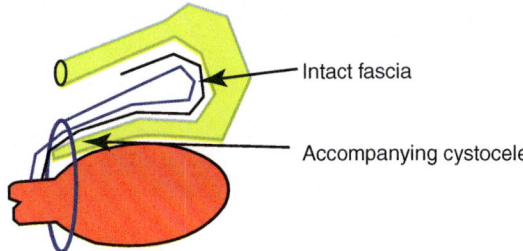

Intact fascia

Accompanying cystocele

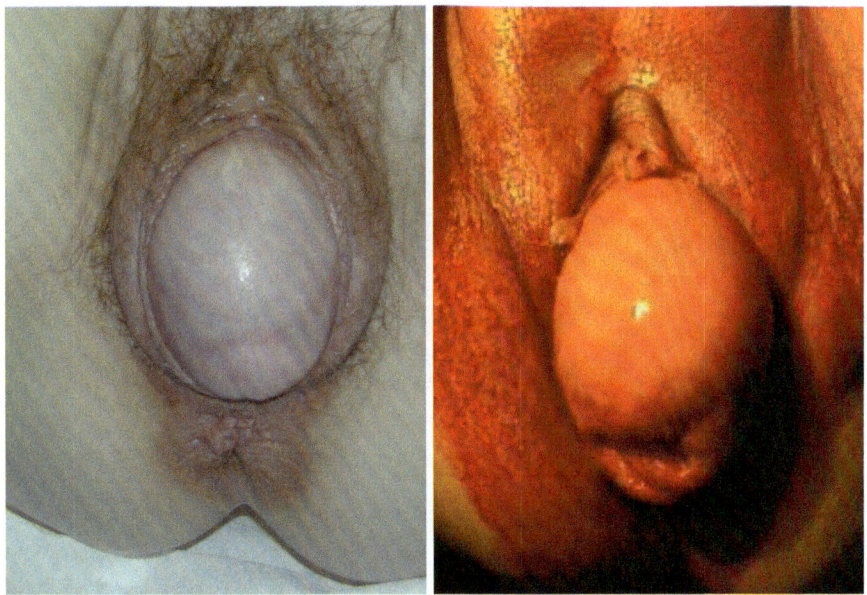

Photos 1 and 2 Central defect: the vaginal wall is smooth and thin (courtesy of Dr. Emmanuel Delorme)

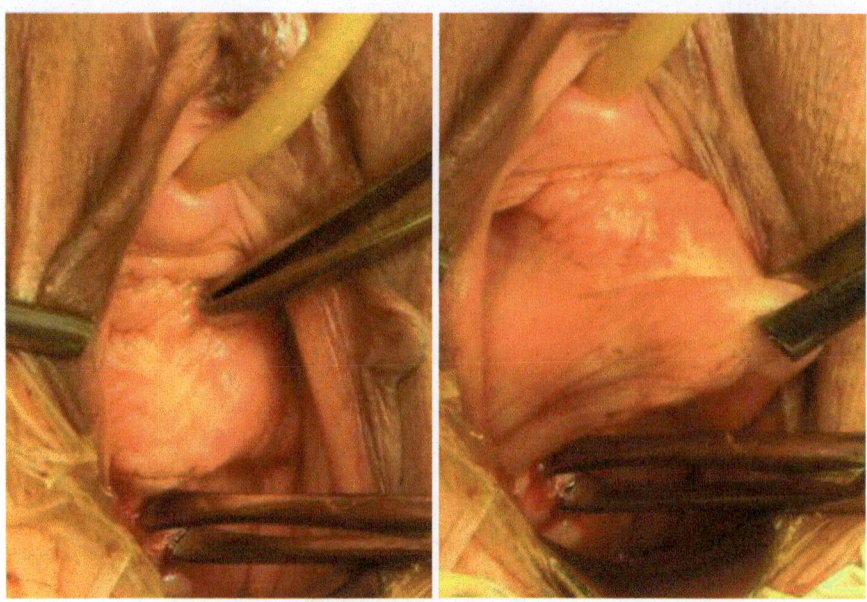

Photos 3 and 4 Lateral defect: the vaginal wall is rough and there are no more lateral gutters (courtesy of Dr. Emmanuel Delorme)

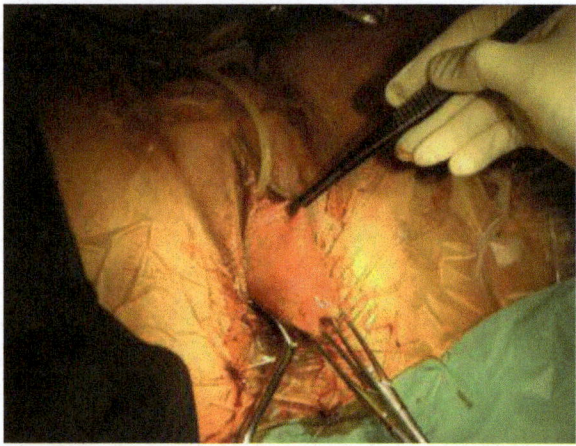

Photo 4 Accompanying cystocele: comes and goes with the descending uterus (courtesy of Dr. Emmanuel Delorme)

3. Level 3 defects concern the lower part of the vagina. Anteriorly, the defect is located on the three distal centimeters of the vagina and in case of defect, a lesion of the pubo-urethral ligament will provoke urethrocele and stress incontinence. Posteriorly, a low rectocele is possible if the perineal body is injured, usually visible at clinical examination because the ano-vulvar distance is diminished less than 1 cm. In both cases, LSCP will not be the correct solution and a vaginal approach should be discussed.

4. Vaginal distension is the visible part of the pathology. Huge distension may sometimes be observed (Photos 1 and 2). It is very similar to scrotal distension in case of inguino scrotal groin hernia in male. As soon as you have treated the hernia, the distension is reversible. Even a large vaginal distension is neither an indication for colpectomy nor a contraindication for LSCP.

3.3 Laparoscopic Anatomy

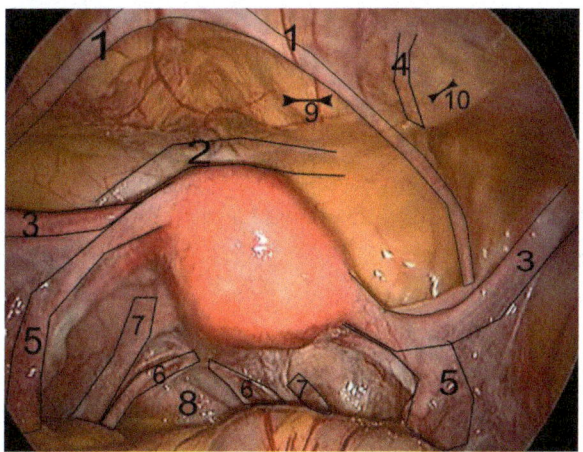

Picture 1 Anatomy (*1* umbilical artery, *2* pubis bone, *3* round ligaments, *4* epigastric vessels, *5* fallopian tubes, *6* utero sacral ligaments, *7* ureters, *8* Douglas pouch, *9* safe place for the 10–12 mm trocar, *10* safe place for the second 5 mm trocar)

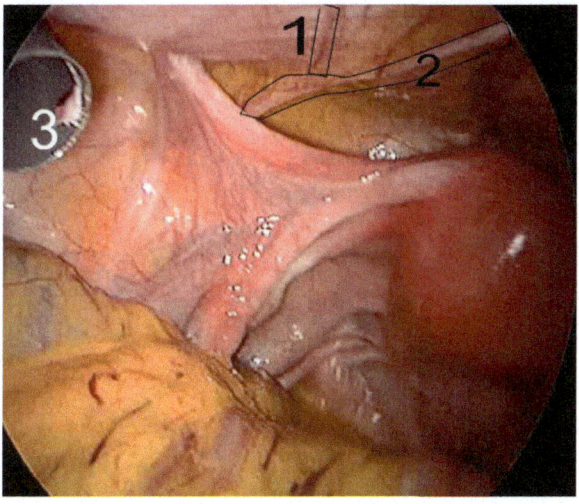

Picture 2 Anatomy (*1* epigastric vessels, *2* umbilical vessels, *3* left lateral trocar)

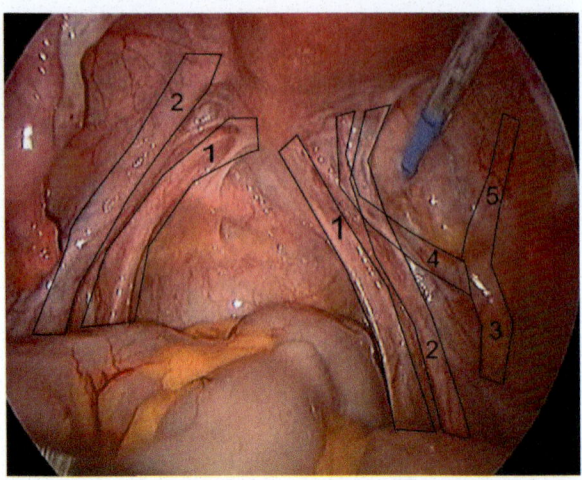

Picture 3 Anatomy (*1* utero sacral ligaments, *2* ureters, *3* hypogastric artery, *4* uterine artery, *5* umbilical artery)

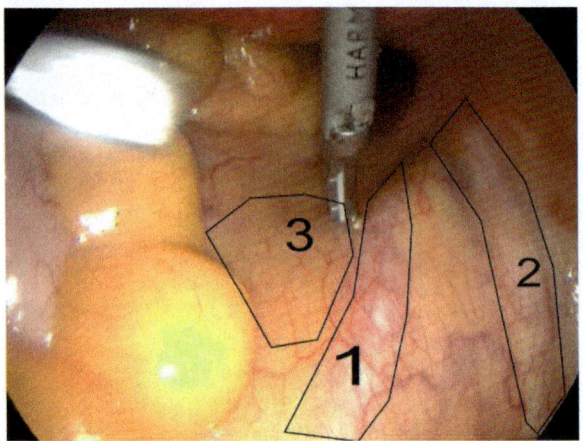

Picture 4 Anatomy (*1* right common iliac artery, *2* right ureter, *3* probable location of the promontory in obese women)

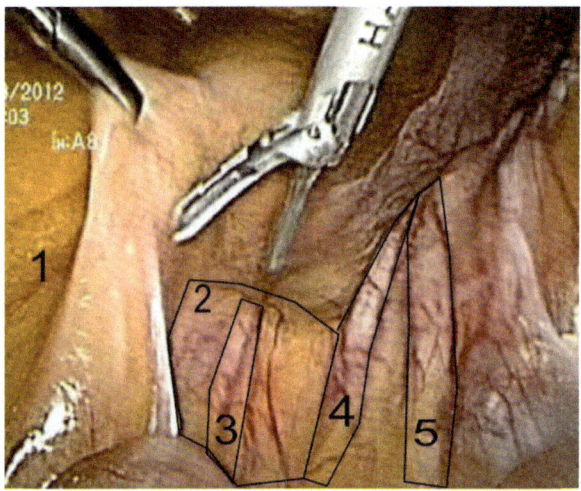

Picture 5 Anatomy (*1* rectum, *2* promontory, *3* medial sacral vein, *4* common iliac artery, *5* ureter crossing the artery in skinny women)

Reference

1. Peter E. Papa, Petros. The Integral Theory System. A simplified clinical approach with illustrative case histories. Pelviperineology 2010;29:37–51. http://www.pelviperineology.org

Operative Technique

4

4.1 Surgical Setting

(a) Uterine mobilization and cul de sac presentation

When the uterus is in place and if you target a conservative surgery, it's crucial to expose correctly the posterior cul de sac of the vagina and to be able to ante-vert and retroflex the uterine body. Several manipulators and cul de sac pre-senter are available on the market. We have chosen the Tintara (Pictures 1 and 2) one because it's cheap, reusable, easy to use and efficient. If not avail-able in your OR, you can replace it with a Leriche retractor (Picture 3) or an equivalent, to present the posterior cul de sac. Then uterine mobilization can be performed by using the disposable and cheap T Lift devices as shown on Pictures 4 and 5.

When the uterus is absent or if you remove it partially or totally during the first step of your procedure, the Leriche retractor (or equivalent) is better than a vaginal tampon because there's no risk to pass a suture or a staple through it.

© Springer International Publishing AG 2017
P. von Theobald, *Laparoscopic Sacrocolpopexy for Beginners*,
DOI 10.1007/978-3-319-57636-7_4

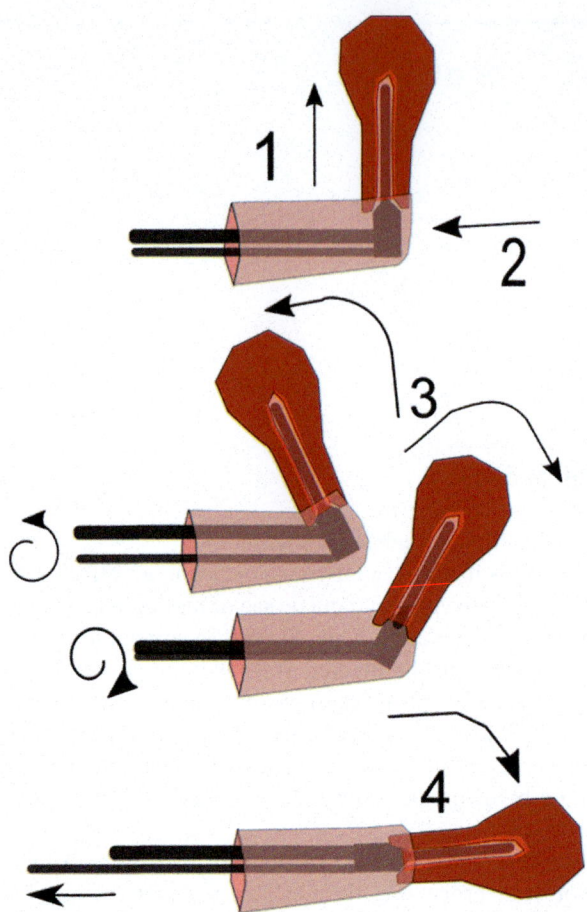

Picture 1 Tintara uterine manipulator (Storz) or Pelosi uterine manipulator (Apple medical). *1* is anteversion of the uterus with presentation of the posterior cul de sac (*2*). *3* is lateral mobilization of the uterus and *4* is retroversion of the uterus

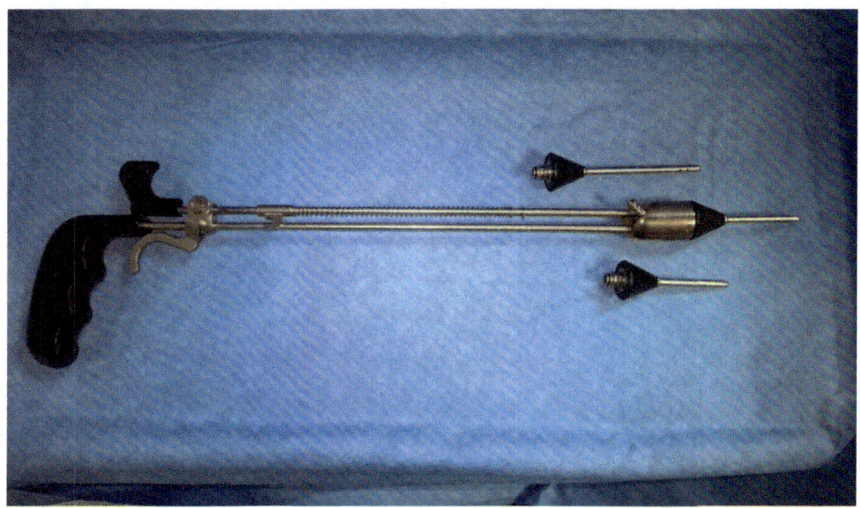

Picture 2 Tintara uterine manipulator (Storz) or Pelosi uterine manipulator (Apple medical)

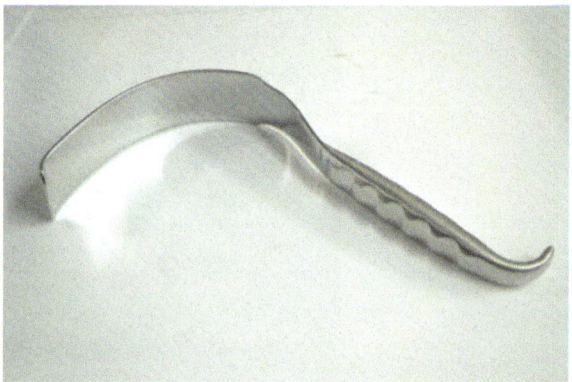

Picture 3 Leriche retractor

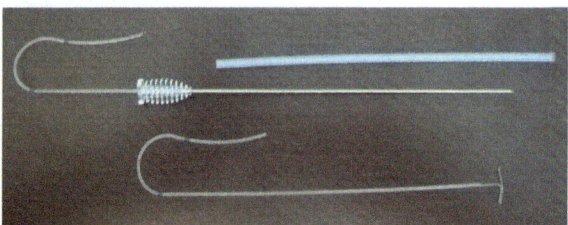

Picture 4 TLift

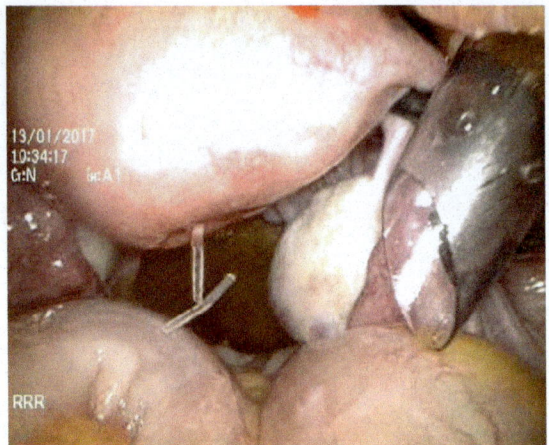

Picture 5 TLift in place to mobilize the uterine body

(b) Trocar setting

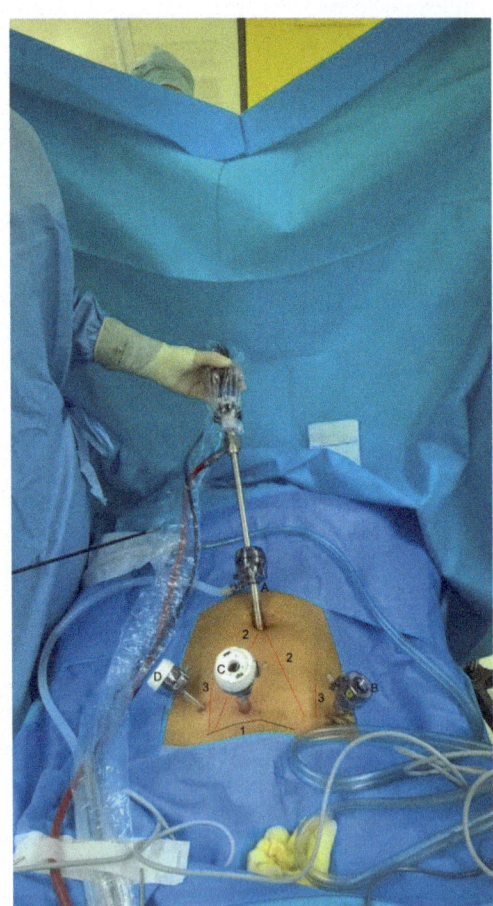

Picture 1 Trocar positioning—*1* is upper limit of pubis bone, *2* is umbilical arteries, *3* is epigastric vessels. Trocar A is in the umbilicus, trocar B is lateral to the left epigastric vessels, trocar C is medial to the right umbilical artery and trocar D is lateral to the right epigastric vessels.

(c) The instruments

No special instruments are required: two atraumatic forceps, two grasping forceps, one scissor, eventually, one needle holder and a suction-irrigation device. Ideally, harmonic scalpel could be used for quick dissection but if not available, a bipolar cautery device can do the job.

4.2   LSCP for Vault Prolapse or After Subtotal Hysterectomy

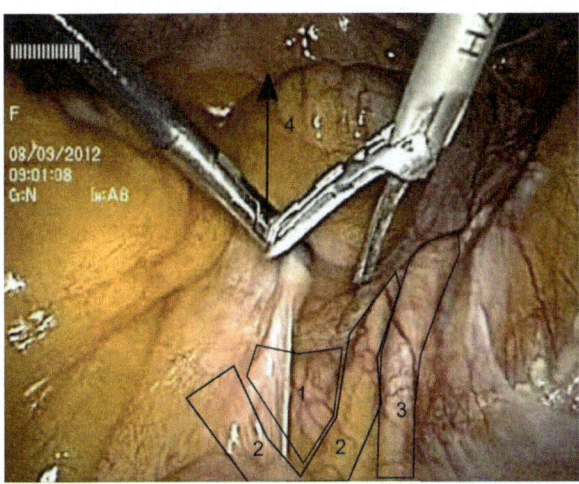

Step 1: Grasp the peritoneum in front of the promontory (*1*) and lift it strongly. The blood vessels (common right iliac artery and vein: *2*) are not adhesive to the peritoneum and your full thickness incision will be safe. Remember: there are two layers to incise; the peritoneum itself and the underlying sheet of fascia. Usually, it is performed in two times. Ureter (*3*) is very distant.

Step 2: The peritoneum is open (two layers) and you can see the extra peritoneal space (*1*) looking like some spider web. You have direct visual access to the promontory (*2*) with the medial sacral vessels that should not be injured (*3*).

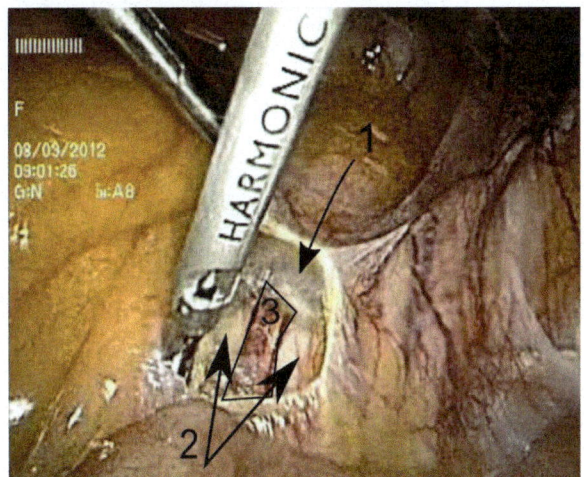

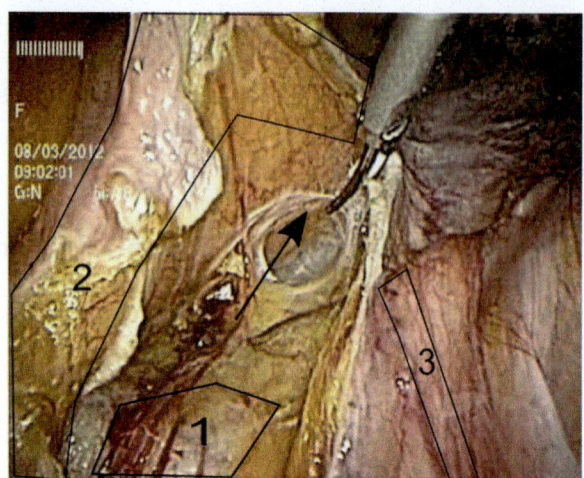

Step 3: The peritoneal opening progresses from the promontory (*1*) towards the Douglas pouch (*arrow*), along the right side of the rectum (*2*), close to the rectum, far from the right ureter (*3*).

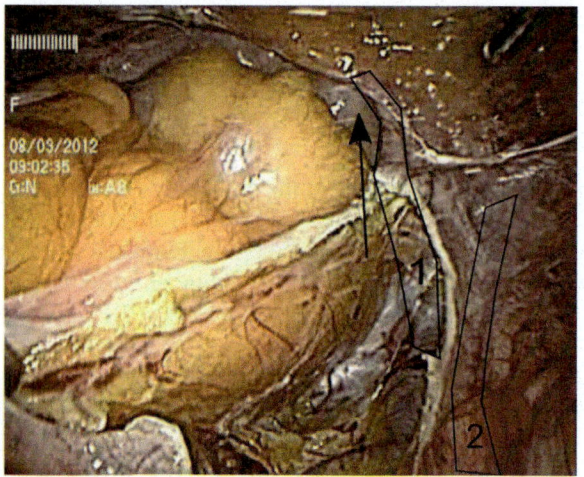

Step 4: The dissection (*arrow*) must stay medial to the uterosacral ligament (*1*). Thus, the extra peritoneal dissection will lead automatically to the rectovaginal wall and stay far from the right ureter (*2*). Always stay close to the rectum.

Step 5: Open (*arrow*) the peritoneum between the rectum (*1*) and the vault (*2*) exposing the pararectal fat. The vault is presented well with the vaginal device. In the pararectal fat, you can frequently see the correct dissection plane to the elevator muscles as a soft spider web area (*3*).

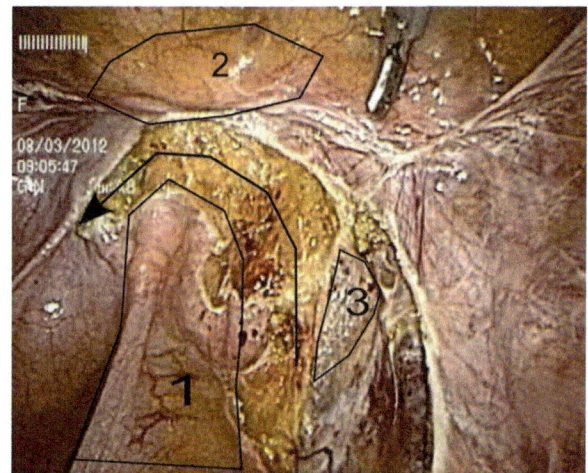

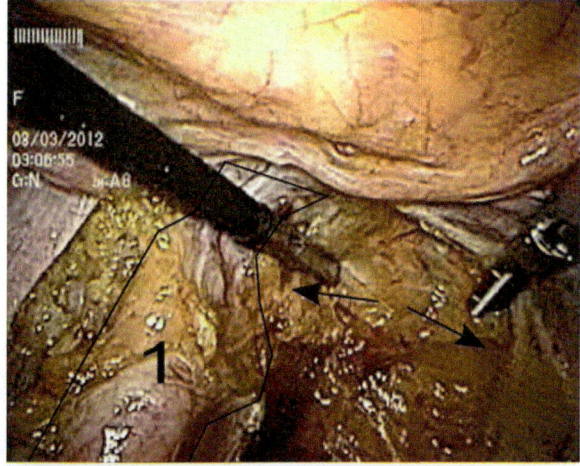

Step 6: Dissect atraumatically, spreading the tissue with the instruments (*arrow*) through the pararectal fat on the right side of the rectum (*1*), guided by the spider web like extraperitoneal adhesion, until you visualize the elevator muscles (*2*).

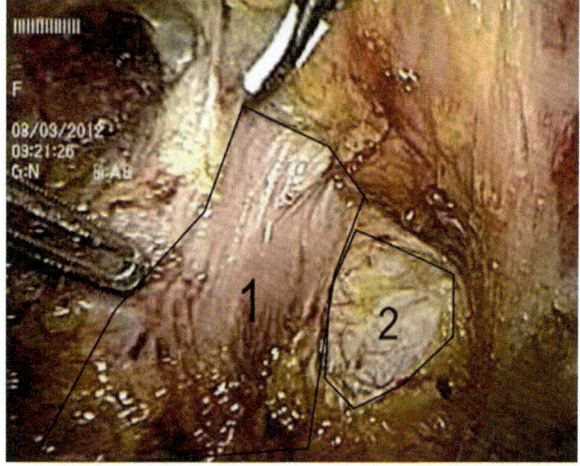

Step 7: Perform the same
dissection on the left.
Rectum (*1*), elevator
muscles (*2*).

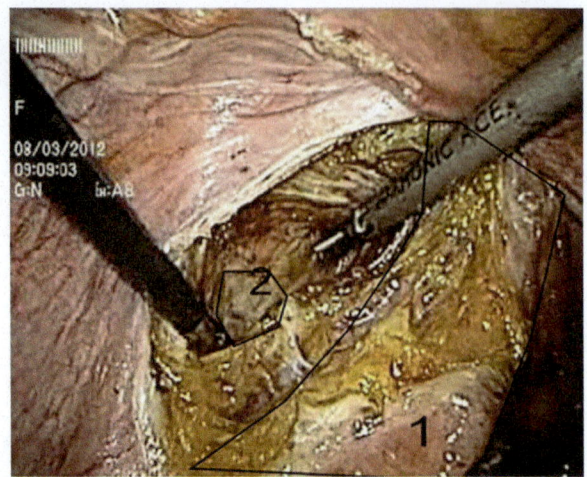

Final view of posterior
dissection. Rectum (*1*),
elevator muscles (*2*).

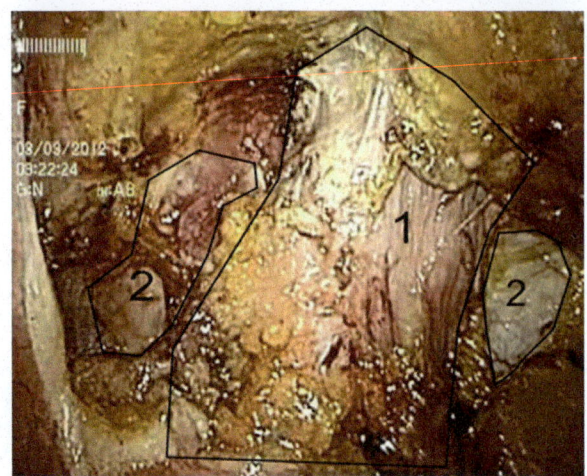

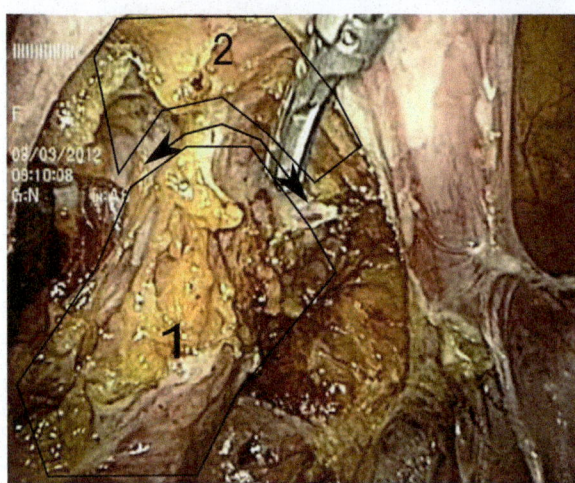

Step 8: Finish opening the
recto (*1*)–vaginal (*2*)
dissection plane (*arrow*).

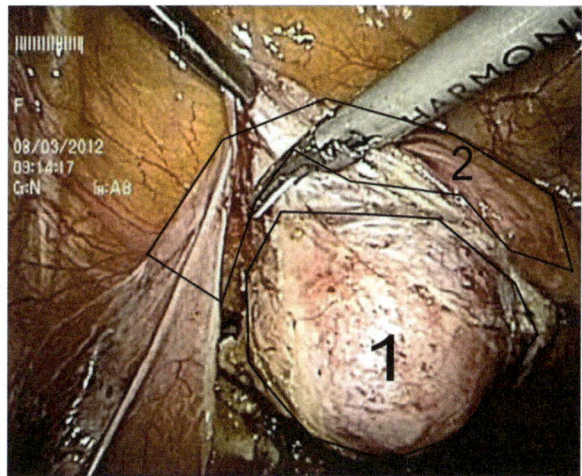

Step 9: Dissect the vault (*1*). All of the peritoneum has to be removed from the vault. Be careful, the bladder (*2*) and the ureters (not visible) are very nearby.

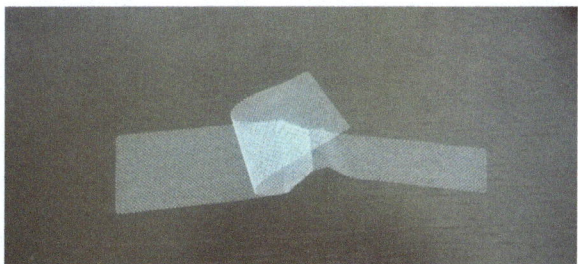

Step 10: Insert the Y shaped mesh through the 10 mm trocar. Either you can use a precut mesh, easily available on the market.

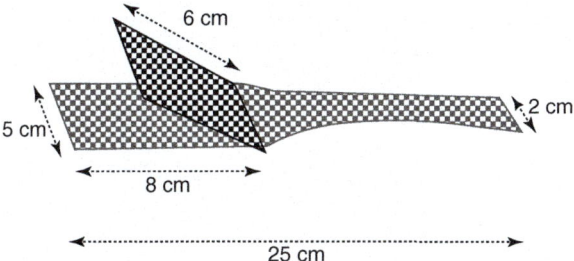

Or you can tailor it yourself from a 30 × 30 cm polypropylene monofilament mesh (it will be much cheaper). In any case, it's crucial to have a mesh that's long enough to reach from the elevator muscles up to the promontory without tension. That means a total length of 20–25 cm. Some precut meshes are only 15 cm long and should always be discarded. If you tailor yourself, just suture anterior and posterior mesh together with some Prolene suture. Shape and dimensions are as follows:

Step 11: Fix the posterior arm of the mesh (*3*) to the elevators (*1*) on both sides of the rectum (*2*).

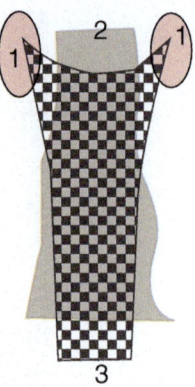

Step 11: This is done here on the right side with staples (EndoHernia 4.4 mm). You can also use sutures (longer and more difficult) or absorbable staples.

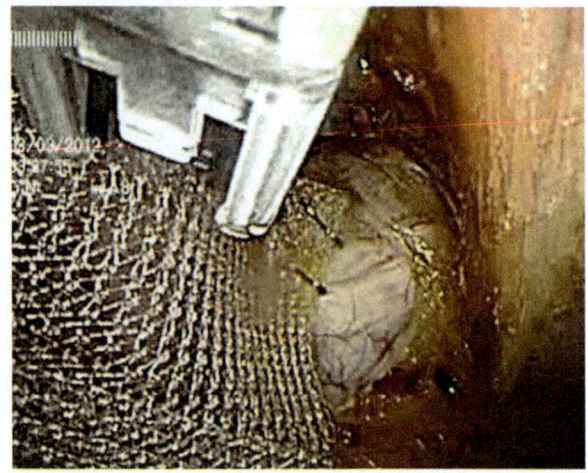

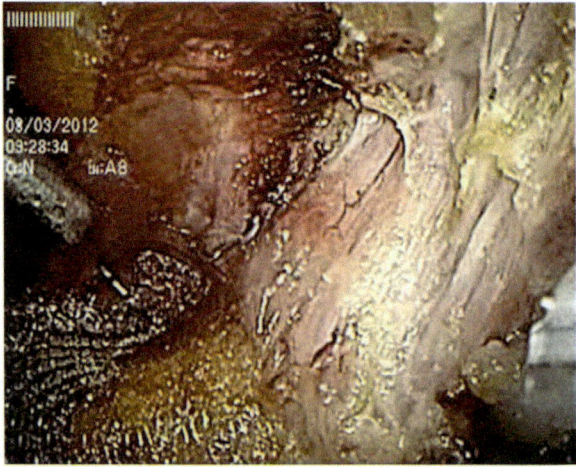

Step 11: Same on the left side.

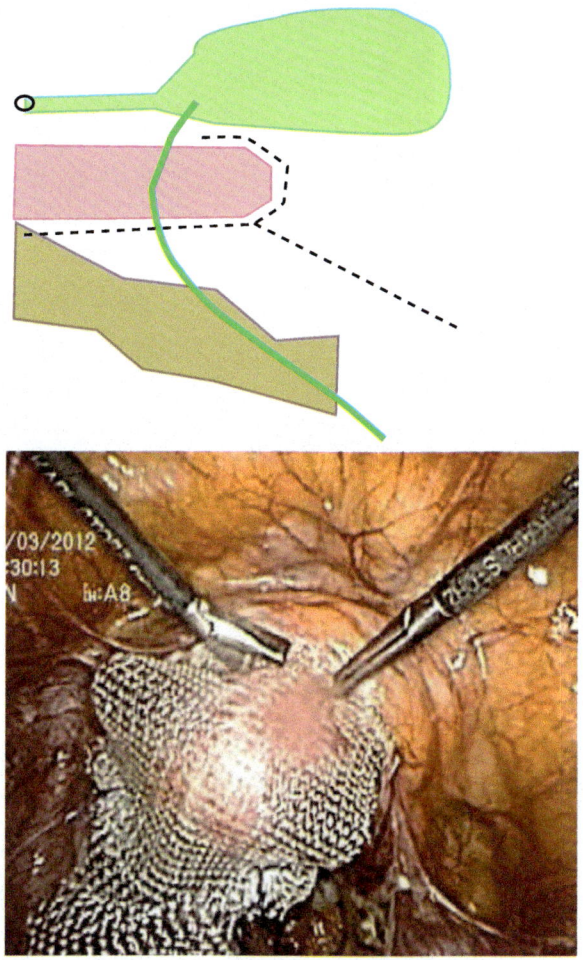

Step 12: Wrap the anterior part of the mesh around the vault.

Step 12: And fix it to the vault. Here, it's performed with metallic staples (endoHernia 4.8 mm) but you can also do it with sutures (absorbable or not)or absorbable staples. About ten staples are requires all around the vault to hold the mesh safely.

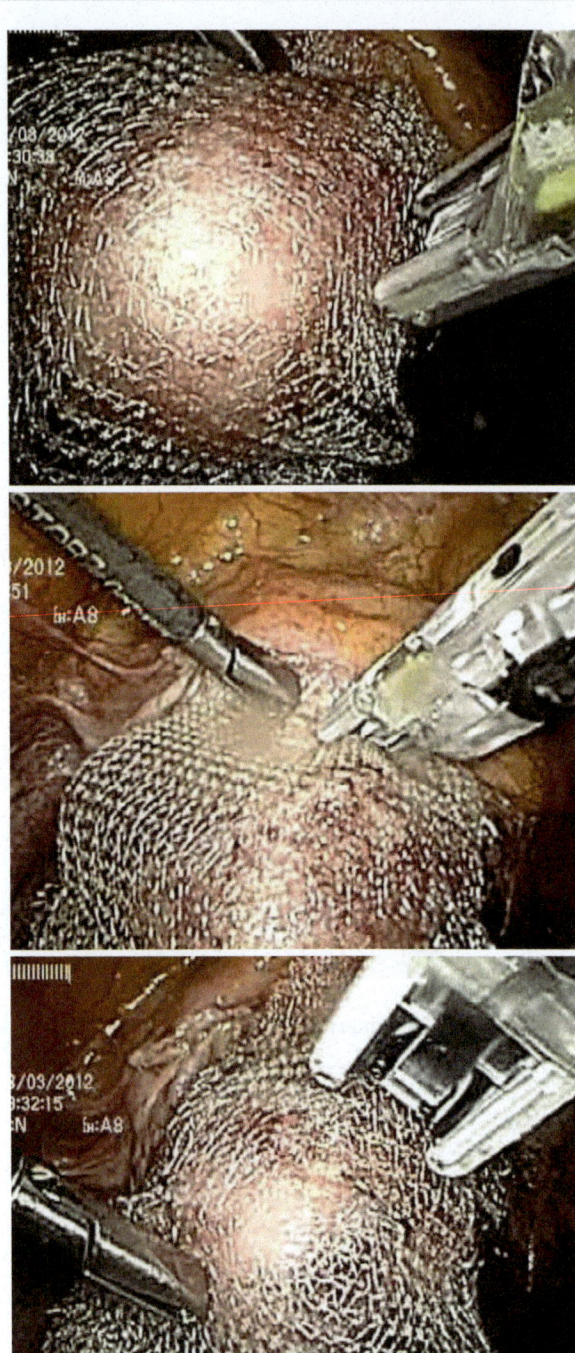

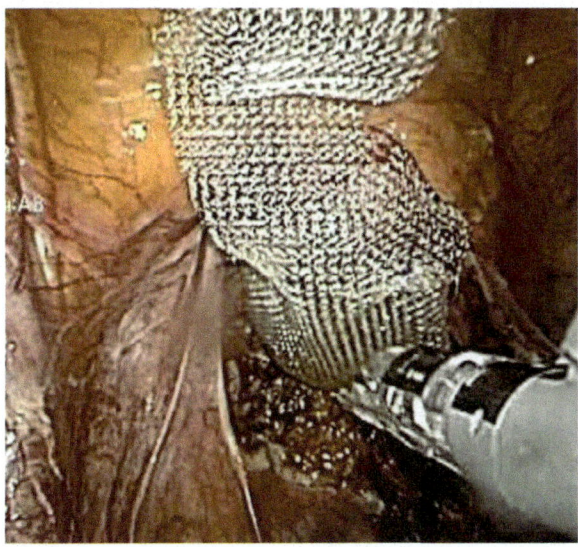

Step 12: The articulated arm of the stapler is a great help to fix the mesh on the posterior part of the vault.

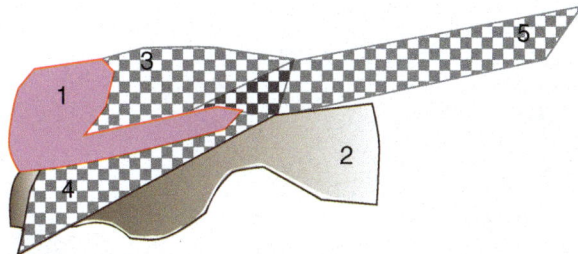

Step 12: The final view before fixation to the promontory. Vault is *1*, rectum is *2*, anterior arm of the mesh is *3* and posterior arm of the mesh is *4*, *5* is the part of the mesh to be attached to the promontory

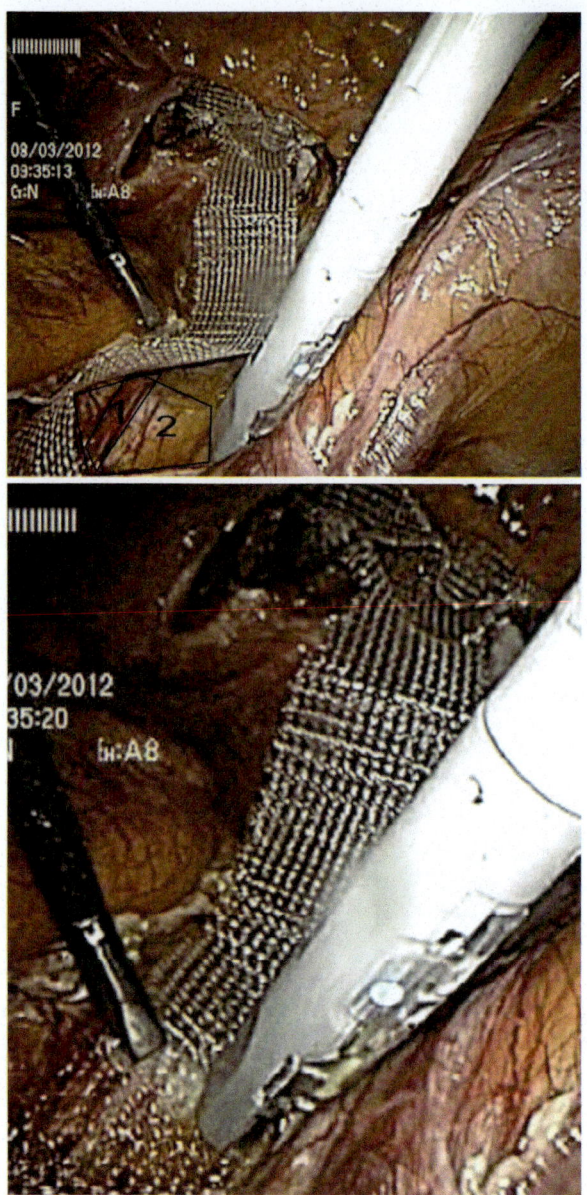

Step 13: Fixation to the promontory **without tension**. *1* is the presacral vessels, *2* is the safe area to fix the mesh with metallic staples (endoHernia 4.0 mm, absorbable staples or sutures (non absorbable monofilament like Prolene should be preferred).

Step 14: Four staples
are set.

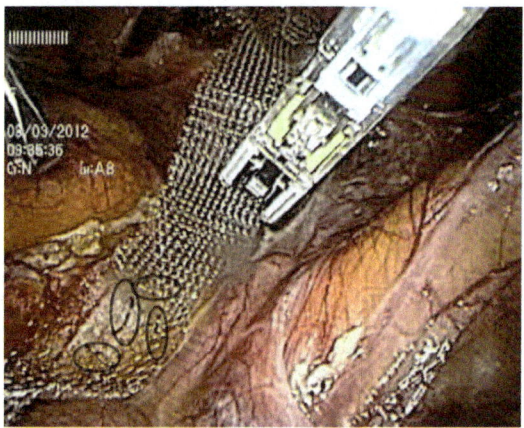

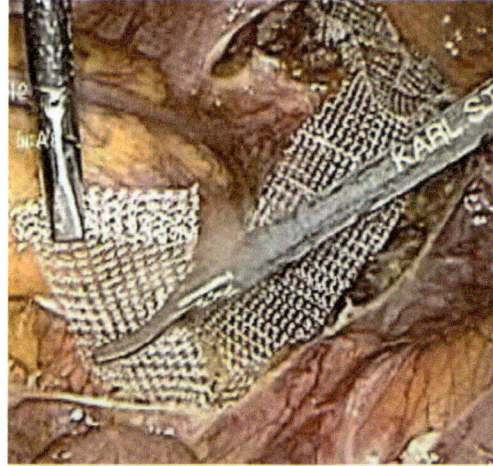

Step 14: Trim the mesh arm and
close the peritoneum. This can be
done with metallic staples
(endoHernia 4.8 mm) as here or
with sutures (auto locking sutures
if available).

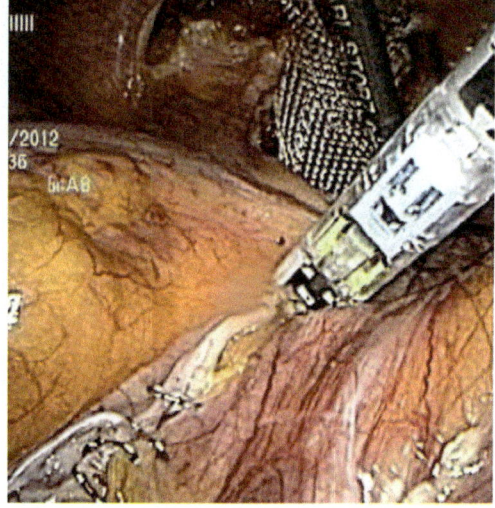

The final aspect. Always
check the ureters in the
end.

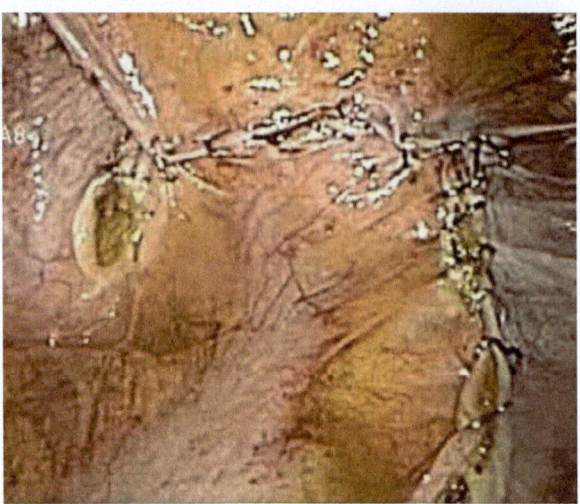

4.3   Conservative LSCP or Laparoscopic Sacrohysteropexy

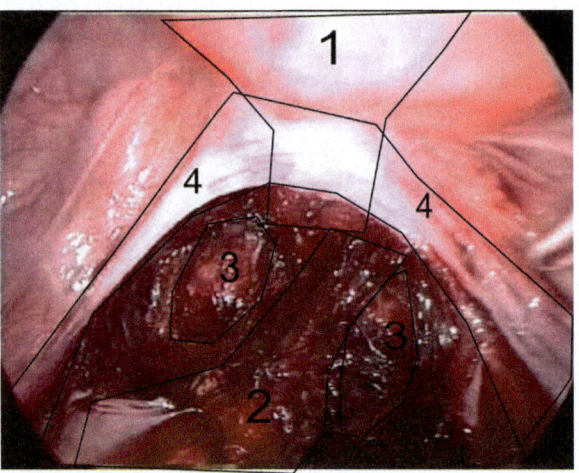

Step 1–8: Dissection of the promontory, opening of the peritoneum, dissection of
the rectovaginal space down to the elevator muscles is identical to the LSCP without
uterus. *1* is uterus, anteverted by the Tintara uterine mobilisator, *2* is dissected
rectum, *3* is elevator muscles and *4* is utero sacral ligaments.

Step 9: Dissection of the bladder. Incise the vesico uterine peritoneum transversally and dissect the bladder from the upper third of the vagina. This dissection is identical to the one used for laparoscopic hyster-ectomy. Don't go too far because the ureters are very close if you get near the trigone. A 4 cm dissection is enough, usually. More may be required in case of anterior vaginal wall distended by a large cystocele.

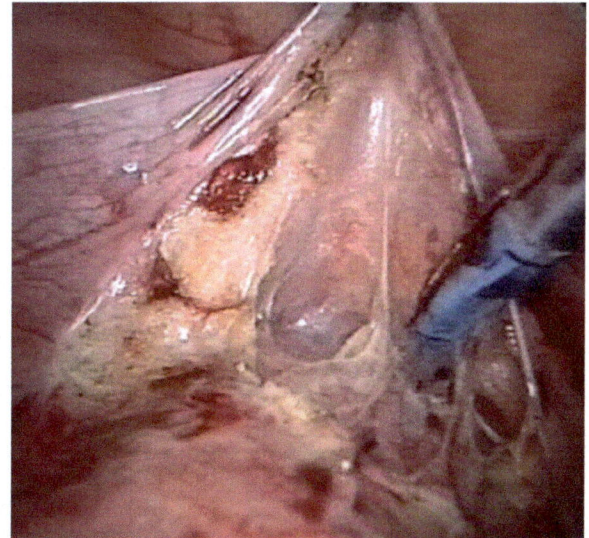

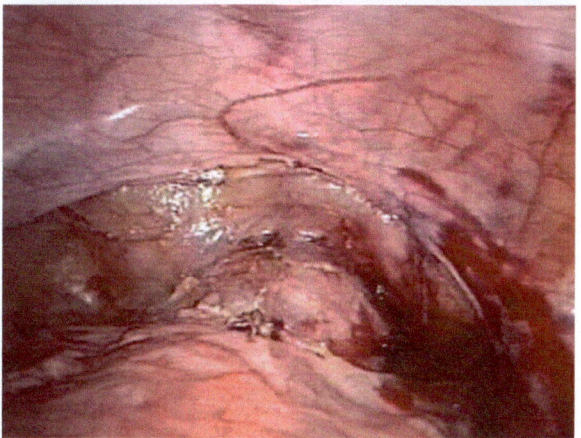

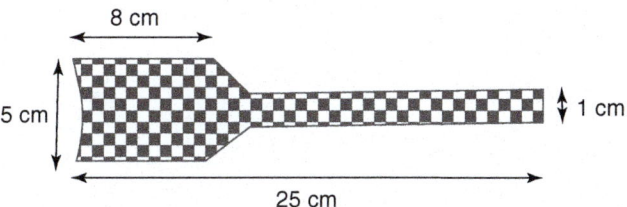

Step 10: Insert the posterior mesh. Here you can see the dimensions of the posterior mesh. It may be pre cut or you can tailor it yourself.

Step 10: Fixation to the elevator muscles is
similar to the technique without uterus. *1* is
elevator muscle, *2* is rectum and *3* is posterior
mesh.

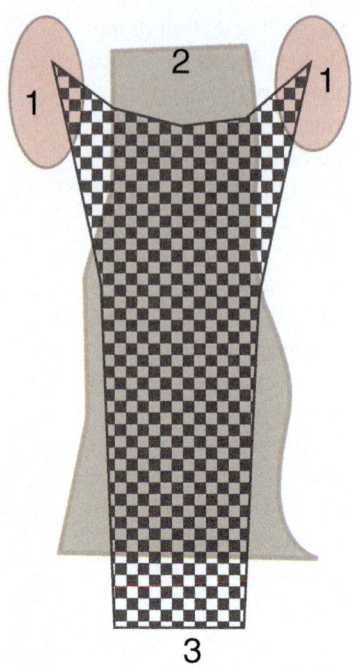

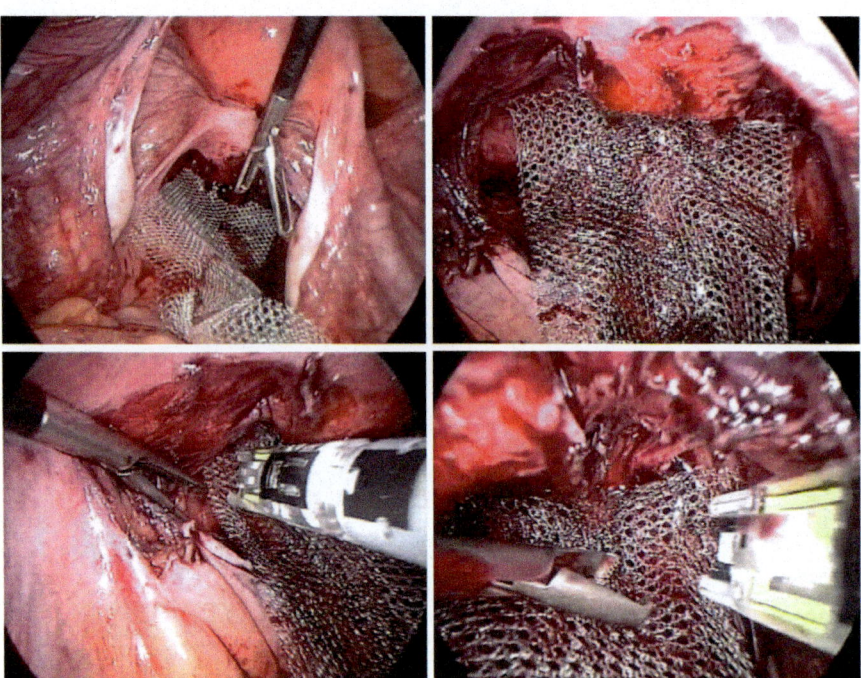

Fixation is here performed with endoHernia 4.8 mm staples but can as well be done
with absorbable or non absorbable sutures or with absorbable staples.

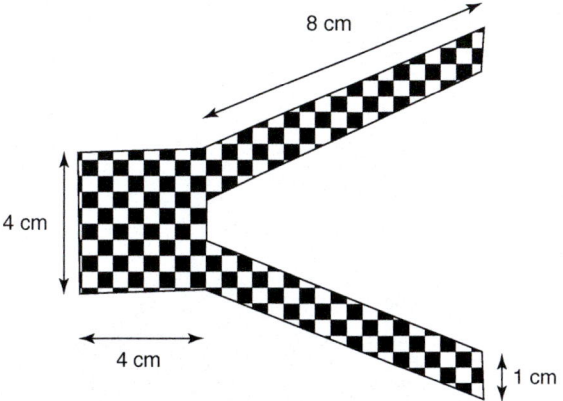

Step 11: Insert the anterior mesh. Dimensions are shown on the drawing. This type of double armed anterior mesh is not available on the market to my knowledge and has to be self tailored. Many surgeons use a single armed mesh, performing the broad ligament only on one side, the right side usually. The double armed mesh has a big advantage; it recreates the pericervical ring and thus, secures the posterior mesh to the uterine isthmus and the posterior vagina without any suture.

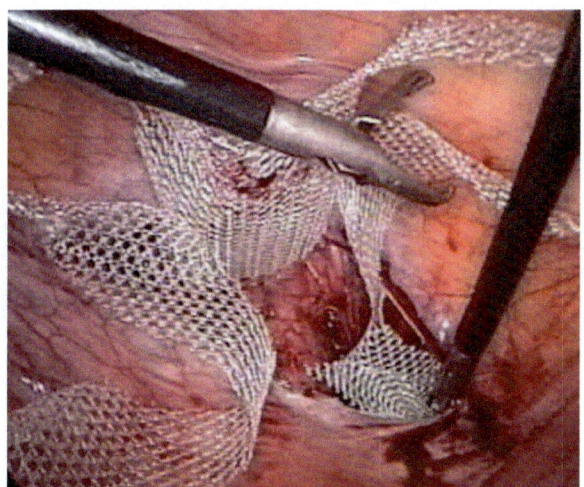

Step 12: Grasp the right arm and insert it in the anterior incision of the right broad ligament. Then antevert the uterus

Step 12: Then antevert
the uterus.

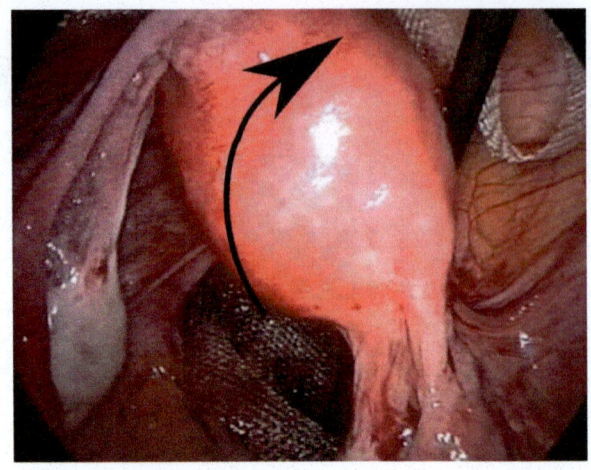

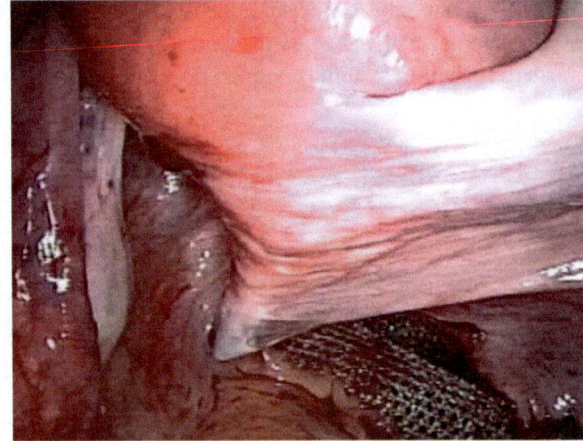

Step 12: And perforate
softly the posterior
sheath to the right broad
ligament. Look for a
vessel free place through
the transparent perito-
neum and push firmly on
the grasper.

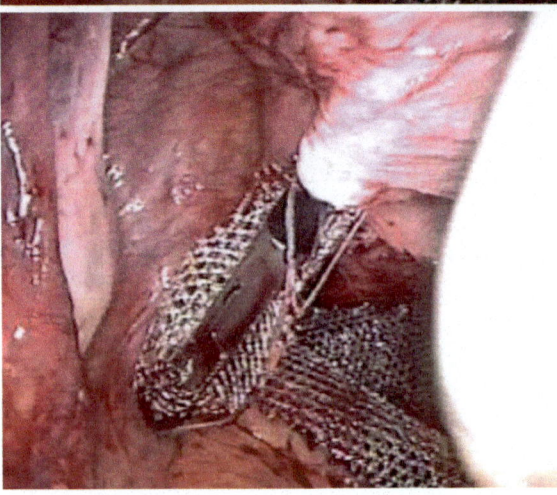

Step 12: Perform the same on the left in order to have one arm passing through the broad ligament on each side.

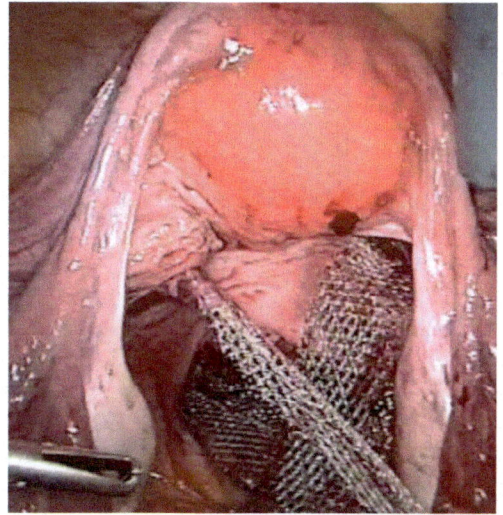

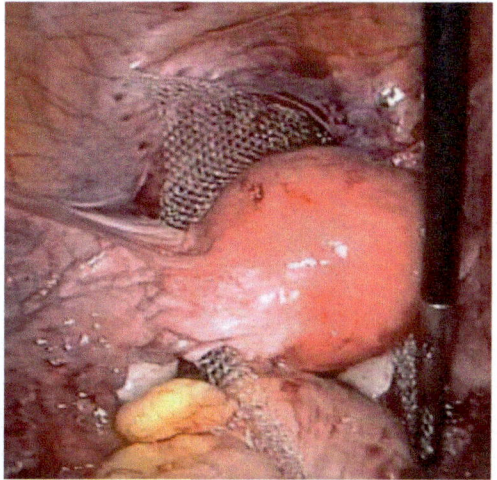

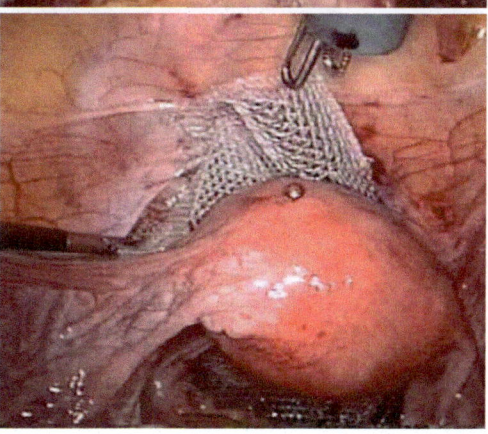

Step 12: Pull on the two arms to place the body of the mesh in the middle.

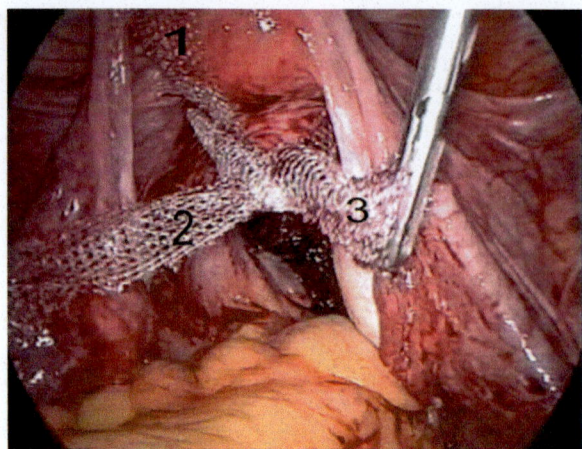

Step 13: Lift the posterior mesh (*1*) and knot the two arms of the anterior mesh (*2* and *3*) together behind the posterior mesh, around the uterine isthmus. No big tension is needed.

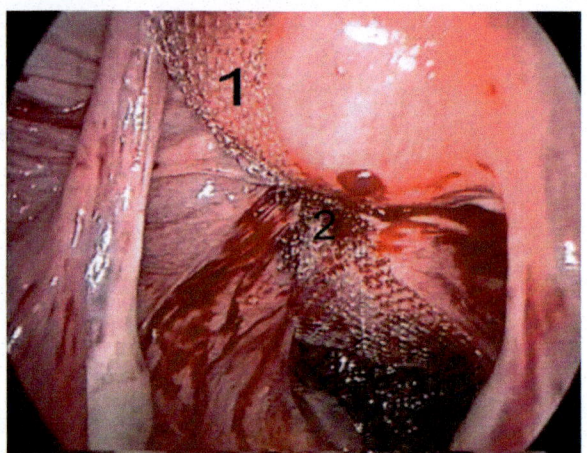

Step 13: Final aspect after trimming of the anterior arms. *1* is posterior mesh, *2* is the knot of the anterior arms.

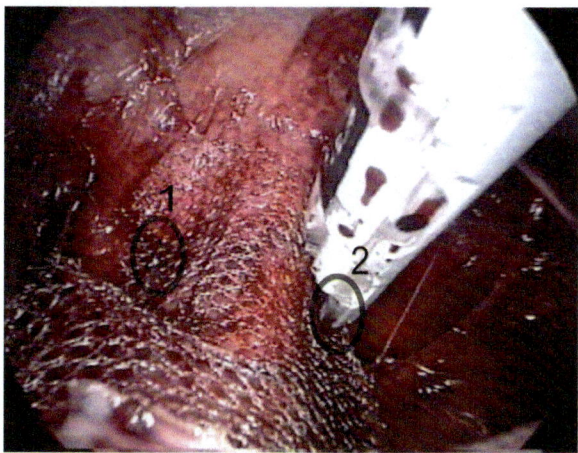

Step 14: Secure the body of the anterior mesh with two staples or two sutures. *1* is left and *2* is right staple to the vagina

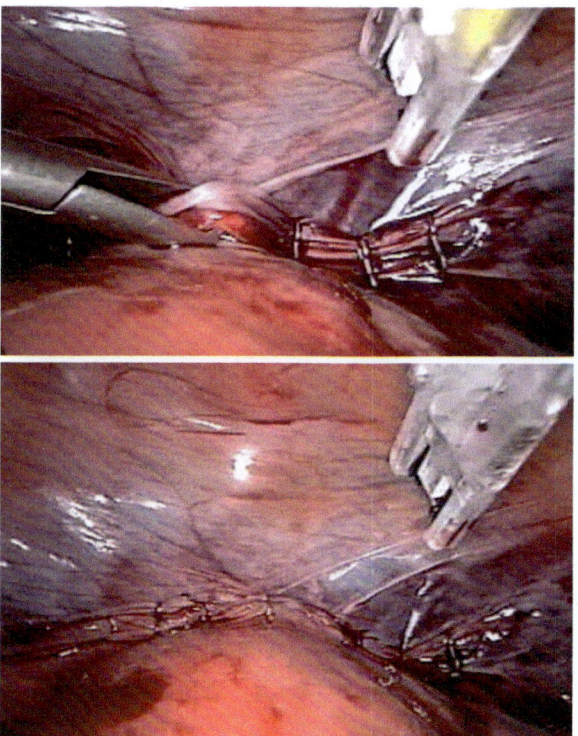

Step 15: Close the vesico uterine peritoneum.

Step 16: Fixation to the
promontory with staples
or sutures: identical to
the technique without
uterus. *1* is vagina, *2* is
rectum, *3* is uterus, *4* is
the posterior mesh.

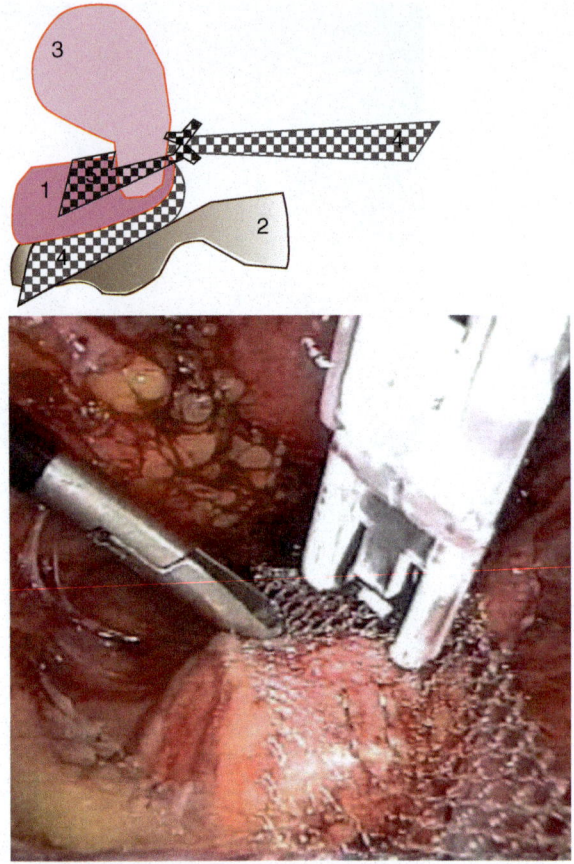

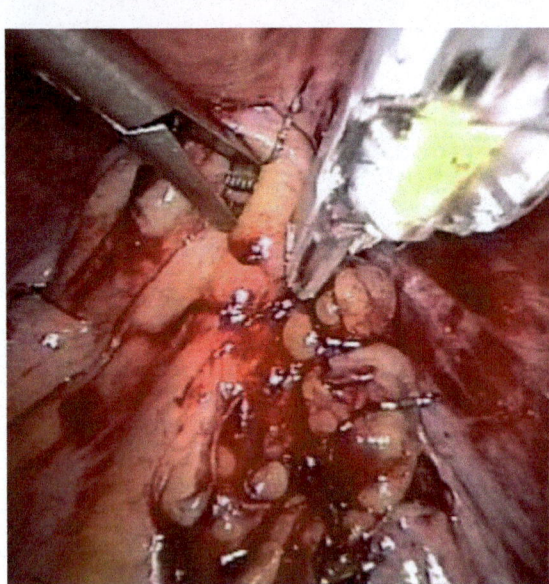

Step 17: Close the
peritoneum as described
previously.

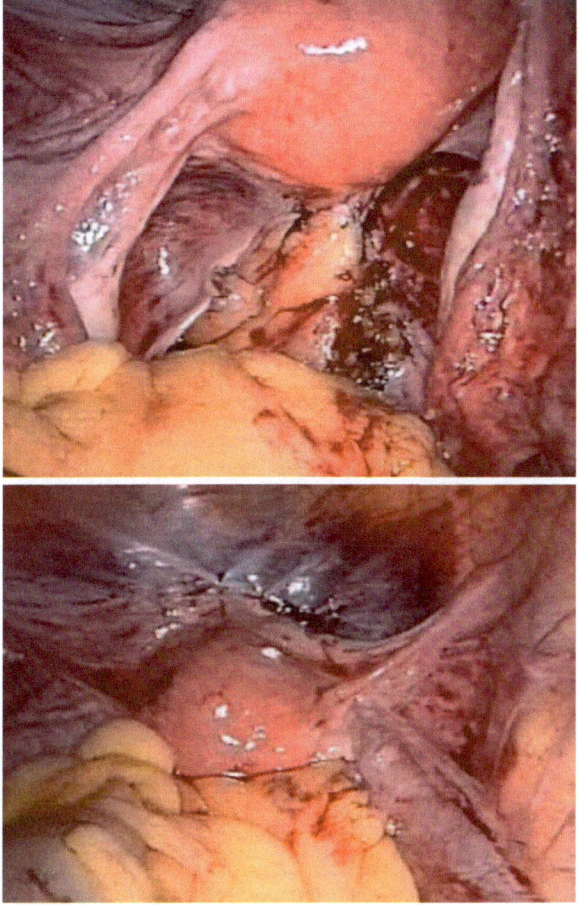

The final aspect. Always check the ureters in the end.

5

Hysterectomy or Not Hysterectomy That Is the Question!

Removing the uterus has been the first treatment for POP performed successfully by vaginal approach in 1521 by Berengarius de-Capri [1]. Since, hysterectomy has become systematic for many authors. Pretty soon, surgeons found out that hysterectomy was not enough to treat POP, replacing a descending uterus with an enterocele. They noticed also that hysterectomy of the non prolapsed uterus was increasing the risk of POP.

At the end of the nineteenth century, dissections showed the crucial role of the fascias and ligaments, especially their pericervical attachments that were playing the role of a keystone. This fact led to the introduction of supracervical hysterectomy (SCH). I will not debate here about the supracervical hysterectomy in general. I just want to explain that it was the best solution for SCP because opening of the vagina (necessary in total hysterectomy) could be avoided as well as the induced complications related to sepsis or mesh erosion.

The debate about hysterectomy or not is not closed. In concerns vaginal as well as abdominal or laparoscopic approach. Of course, in some patients, hysterectomy is mandatory: lesions of the cervix (CIN 2 or 3), adenomyosis, symptomatic myomas, hypertrophic uterine body or cervix, atypical lesions of the endometrium, etc. For the other patients, there are many pros and cons for systematic supracervical hysterectomy (SCH) during LSCP. Let's have a look at the main of them.

5.1 The Pros

(a) **SCH facilitates the procedure**. Right, the mesh is easier to apply because you don't have to channelize the broad ligament. Thus, you take no risk of injuring the uterine vessels. On the other hand, you have to do the SCH and morcellate the uterine body. This makes the procedure more sophisticated.

(b) **SCH avoids a further hysterectomy that might be difficult.** Right and wrong. Yes, you will never have to perform hysterectomy, but in case of bleeding, adenomyosis or HPV related lesions, you may have to remove the cervix, which is

© Springer International Publishing AG 2017
P. von Theobald, *Laparoscopic Sacrocolpopexy for Beginners*,
DOI 10.1007/978-3-319-57636-7_5

much more difficult, because the mesh is sutured to it. In fact, having personally performed more than 20 laparoscopic hysterectomies (including three Wertheim operations for cervical cancer), after SCP or LSCP, I noticed that this procedure was not to be feared. Adhesions are usually very tiny after LSCP. The mesh is easy to visualize. The right ureter is frequently very close to the mesh and has to be properly dissected. Then the mesh can be cut close to the uterine isthmus and the rest of the operation is identical to the hysterectomy in the non operated patients. Careful closure of the vagina has to be performed in order to avoid any extrusion of the remaining synthetic mesh. It is advisable after vaginal closure to suture the distal and proximal parts of the mesh together in order to avoid a further vault prolapse. If the cervix has to be removed, vaginal extra peritoneal approach is still possible and advisable.

(c) **SCH improves the results**. Very difficult to say if right or wrong. There are no randomized series, only retrospective studies [2]. Most of these papers show no significant difference in the functional or anatomical results between LSCP patients with or without hysterectomy. There is probably a selection bias in these retrospective series because in current practice, when the uterus is big, myomatous, it is usually removed. It is very difficult to access the rectovaginal space if the uterus is large sized. Further, a very heavy uterus may put the meshes under tension, inducing pain and, maybe, suture disruption.

5.2   The Cons

(a) **SCH makes the procedure much longer**. Right, because you have to add to your LSCP (1–4 h in literature, see Chap. 8), the duration of the SCH with morcellation (1.5–2 h in literature). This gives you a 4–6 h procedure under general anesthesia. If you use our tips and tricks and if you have completed your learning curve, it may take only 2–3 h, which seems much more acceptable.

(b) **SCH necessitates a morcellator**. Right, unless you perform a mini-laparotomy or a vaginal incision in the posterior cul de sac to extract the uterine body. In the first case, it cannot any longer be considered as a laparoscopic SCP, and you lose many advantages of minimal invasive surgery in terms of post operative pain, esthetics and risk of adhesions. In the second case, you lose the theoretical advantage of not opening the vagina. Opening the vagina is supposed to provoke a higher rate of sepsis and mesh erosions [3, 4]. The use of a morcellator has recently raised a huge debate about the risk of spreading malignant tissue during morcellation, mainly endometrial cancer (which should be detected before POP repair), and myometrial occult sarcoma. In a very recent study, the overall prevalence of occult malignancy within morcellated specimens was 0.5% [5], mainly undiagnosed endometrial carcinoma.

(c) **SCH increases the risk of intraoperative complications**. Right. For instance, the monopolar loop or the monopolar hook used to cut the uterine isthmus is at high risk of injuring the bowel or the bladder in untrained hands. Many case reports of bowel injury due to the morcellator are reported in literature.

Conclusion

We could argue about this subject during pages, give hundreds of references in literature without coming to an end. Hysterectomy, supracervical if possible, should be decided according to the clinical needs first (big uterus, cervical, endo or myometrial lesion) and according to the patient's wishes. There is no systematic attitude and every individual case has to be discussed. One main principle: "primum non nocere". A useless procedure can only induce complications and bring no benefit. On the other hand, an incomplete procedure, related to insufficient skill or equipment, may reduce intra operative complications but will finish with a poor clinical result. My personal opinion is that too many useless hysterectomies are performed all over the world. In my own series between 1993 and 2002 [6], only 5% of patients underwent concomitant SCH. Today, I would probably double this rate. You have to consider that correct and easily available morcellators appeared on the market only in the late nineties. In my early experience, morcellation was performed with scissors or a blunt scalpel introduced into the abdominal cavity. Such conditions may influence the decisions. Conditions may also change in future with new technology.

References

1. Emge LA, Durfee RB. Pelvic organ prolapse: four thousand years of treatment. Clin Obstet Gynecol. 1996;9:997–1032.
2. Pan K, Cao L, Ryan NA, Wang Y, Xu H. Laparoscopic sacral hysteropexy versus laparoscopic sacrocolpopexy with hysterectomy for pelvic organ prolapse. Int Urogynecol J. 2016 Jan;27(1):93–101.
3. Myers EM, Siff L, Osmundsen B, Geller E, Matthews CA. Differences in recurrent prolapse at 1 year after total vs supracervical hysterectomy and robotic sacrocolpopexy. Int Urogynecol J. 2015 Apr;26(4):585–9.
4. Crane AK, Geller EJ, Sullivan S, Robinson BL, Myers EM, Horton C, Matthews CA. Short-term mesh exposure after robotic sacrocolpopexy with and without concomitant hysterectomy. South Med J. 2014 Oct;107(10):603–6.
5. Vallabh-Patel V, Saiz C, Salamon C, Francis A, Pagnillo J, Culligan P. Prevalence of occult malignancy within morcellated specimens removed during laparoscopic sacrocolpopexy. Female Pelvic Med Reconstr Surg. 2016 Jul–Aug;22(4):190–3.
6. Massou E, Chéret A, Marcus-Braun N, von Theobald P. Laparoscopic sacro(hystero)colpopexy: twenty years after. Women's Health & Gynecology. 2016 Apr 7. http://scientonline.org/open-access/laparoscopic-sacrohysterocolpopexy-twenty-years-after.pdf

Stress Urinary Incontinence (SUI) Cure Procedure at the Time of the LSCP or Not?

6

This is also a very old debate, still open, and not only concerning laparoscopic repair of POP, but any technique. In our early experience in the 90s, we tried to reproduce exactly what was done with laparotomy. At that time, the rule in Europe was to perform a Burch colposuspension systematically at the time of SCP except when the patient had had it previously. I just want to remind you that Burch colposuspension was known to induce enteroceles in a high rate of cases and these enteroceles required SCP to be cured. This sequence was not rare. Later on, we stopped performing SUI repair procedures in patients who had neither symptomatic nor occult SUI.

At the end of the 90s, Burch colposuspension was quickly replaced by vaginal suburethral slings of various kinds: TVT, TOT, minislings. Thus, performing the whole procedure through the same laparoscopic approach was not possible anymore and all urogynecologists had to become vaginal surgeons for SUI repair.

Three recent publications summarize the state of art in 2016.

Salerno in 2016 [1] selects patients as we do, according to a preoperative stress test into three groups: SUI, occult SUI and negative stress test. The first two undergo a sling operation. He finds that SUI was cured in 77% of patients of the first two groups and de novo SUI appeared in 19% of the non sling patients. De novo urge incontinence appeared in respectively 9%, 15% and 19% of patients of each group. Quality of life questionnaires UDI-6 and UIQ-7 improve in all groups after 3 years of follow up. The authors feel happy with these results and estimate that their strategy is correct.

Jeon [2] published in 2014 the results of a big observational cohort of 223 patients assigned to a sling or non sling group in the same way. Their results and conclusions are almost opposite. After 2 years of follow up, 5.4% of the sling group and 28.6% of the non sling group had SUI. Their conclusion is that a prolapse reduction stress test is not sufficient to determine the need for an anti SUI procedure at the time of SCP.

van der Ploeg [3] published in 2014 a meta analysis including seven trials on the subject. He found a high clinical and statistical heterogeneity and conclusions were

© Springer International Publishing AG 2017
P. von Theobald, *Laparoscopic Sacrocolpopexy for Beginners*,
DOI 10.1007/978-3-319-57636-7_6

hard to draw. In women with symptomatic SUI before POP repair, no significant difference between sling and no sling group could be found, amazingly. In asymptomatic women, combination surgery resulted in a significant lower incidence of subjective de novo SUI but the difference was not significant for objective de novo SUI. In the group of patients with occult SUI before POP repair, the occurrence of post operative objective SUI was significantly reduced in the sling group with a RR = 0.4. Interesting was the fact that adverse events and prolonged catheterization occurred more frequently in the sling group, but mainly after vaginal POP repair. He concluded that combination surgery reduces the risk of post operative SUI but may increase the risk of some complications.

As you see, the debate is still open. The series are not easily comparable and there's no well led randomized trial comparing results with or without combined sling in all groups of patients undergoing LSCP. Our advice is to insert a sling concomitantly in patients with symptomatic or occult SUI.

References

1. Salerno J, de Tayrac R, Droupy S, Costa P, Llinares E, Fatton B, Wagner L. Impact of laparoscopic sacrocolpopexy, with or without a midurethral sling, on lower urinary tract symptoms. Prog Urol. 2016 Jun;26(7):401–8.
2. Jeon MJ, Kim JY, Moon YJ, Bai SW, Yoo EH. Two-year urinary outcomes of sacrocolpopexy with or without transobturator tape: results of a prolapse-reduction stress test-based approach. Int Urogynecol J. 2014 Nov;25(11):1517–22.
3. van der Ploeg JM, van der Steen A, Oude Rengerink K, van der Vaart CH, Roovers JP. Prolapse surgery with or without stress incontinence surgery for pelvic organ prolapse: a systematic review and meta-analysis of randomized trials. BJOG. 2014 Apr;121(5):537–47.

How to Start with LSCP When You're a Beginner?

In this section of the book, I want to help beginners to move progressively towards their first LSCP without stress. To reach that goal, some basic skills are to be learnt as a prerequisite.

7.1   Step One: Basic Skills

(a) Techniques of pneumoperitoneum and trocar introduction. A basic training in laparoscopy, as taught to every resident in surgery or gynecology, is mandatory. Safety maneuvers, different techniques to establish safely a pneumoperitoneum, correct insertion of the trocars are the first step to learn laparoscopy. Simple procedures like tubal ligation, blue dye testing, ovarian cystectomy, will help the student to master the basic gestures on the patient, usually under supervision by a senior laparoscopist.

(b) Training on laparotrainer. This kind of training, usually organized in sessions by universities or scientific societies, is crucial to master quickly the 2D vision and the main gestures like grasping and moving items, dissecting structures and suturing techniques. Having mentored laparoscopic trainings on simulators since 1988, I can say that it takes no more than 20 h of work on a laparotrainer to be able to master sutures and knots at a reasonable speed (pictures below)

© Springer International Publishing AG 2017   51
P. von Theobald, *Laparoscopic Sacrocolpopexy for Beginners*,
DOI 10.1007/978-3-319-57636-7_7

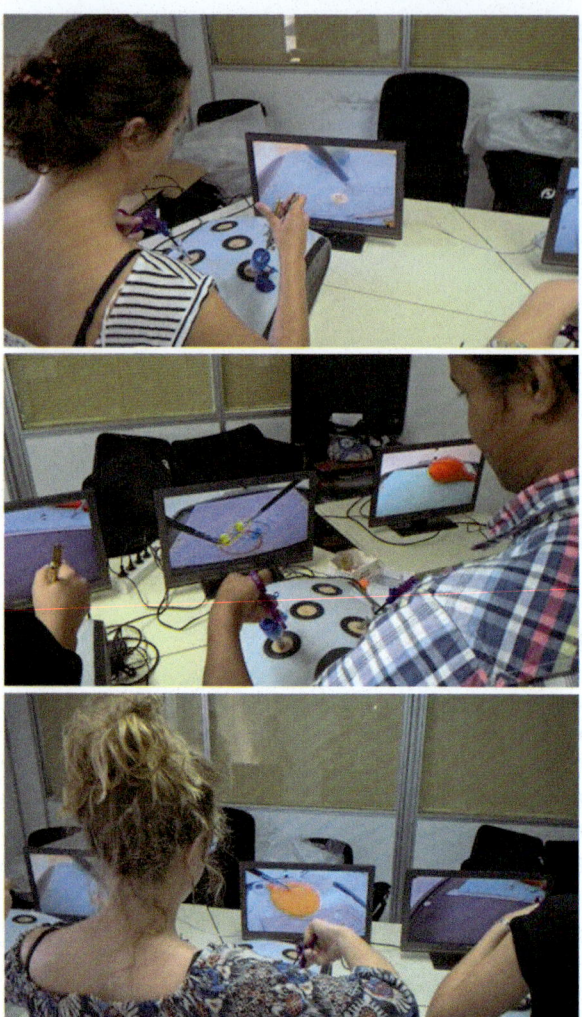

Pictures: Simulation in laparoscopy

(c) Anatomy. Perfect knowledge of the pelvic anatomy is necessary before starting LSCP. Knowledge of the position of pelvic blood vessels, ligaments and fascias, anatomy of the rectum and of the bladder, limits of the pararectal and paravesical spaces, course of the ureters, is essential before starting to perform the first LSCP. Anatomy can be learnt in book or in interactive 3D DVDs. It can also be learnt during live laparoscopy or on cadaver dissection.

7.2   Step Two: Total Laparoscopic Hysterectomy

Total laparoscopic hysterectomy (THL) is an operation that involves almost every skill needed for LSCP. Spend some more attention and time on some specific steps of the procedure in order to prepare you for LSCP. Dissection of the bladder is very similar to the anterior dissection during LSCP and appears as an excellent training. Try to dissect the bladder low enough to see the bare white vaginal wall over a length of 3 or 4 cm and try to localize the ureters laterally. Posterior dissection may also be a good training if you open the peritoneum between the vagina and the rectum before cutting the uterosacral ligaments. You will see the rectovaginal space opening under the pressure of the CO_2 and the white posterior wall of the vagina will be visible over a couple of centimeters. Spotting the ureters on the pelvic sidewalls is also a very useful exercise, especially in overweighed patients, in which the fatty tissue is frequently hiding these structures, forcing you to open the peritoneum and dissect the extra peritoneal space to localize them. In the end, suturing the vaginal cuff is another useful exercise to your laparoscopic skills. Try to do it in different ways: extra peritoneal knots, intra peritoneal knots, running sutures. Mastering THL is crucial; the learning curve takes 30–50 patients. Then you can start to plan your first LSCP.

Of course, for surgeons that are not gynecologists and who don't perform hysterectomies, this step doesn't exist and they'll have to move directly towards step 3.

7.3   Step Three: Watch the Others

It is very important to see the technique performed by trained surgeons who do it as a routine. And watching videos is insufficient to learn because on a video, that usually lasts about 10–20 min, only successful gestures are shown. No difficulty or issue appears on the film. It is crucial to see complete procedures to become able to face any situation. Many national or international meetings program live surgery sessions in which the operation is commented by a moderator and questions may be asked. Another way to see live operations is to be invited into the OR by a trained colleague and, if you're lucky, to assist him during the operation. This is even better than live sessions during congresses because you can see how the OR is organized. You see all the instruments, how they are handled by the surgeon and by the nurses. The information shared is more intimate and you will be more likely to learn some tips and tricks that the surgeon has made up to simplify the operation. It also establishes links that may help you further to start a kind of mentorship that is very useful to start LSCP. The ideal mentorship would be to go to the mentor and watch a couple of LSCP performed by him, then to schedule two LSCP in your own OP and to invite your mentor. He performs the first LSCP with you as an assistant and you perform the second with him assisting you. It is certainly difficult to organize but, in our experience, it is the best way to start quickly and safely.

Our advice is to see at least 5–10 procedures before starting. It is very important to start quickly after having seen the operations; in our experience, if you don't start within 3 or 4 months, you will not start at all.

7.4   Step Four: The Very First LSCP. Don't Stress, You're Ready

1. Follow the check list:

   You know perfectly the anatomy.

   You have performed a lot of laparoscopies before, including sutures, retro-peritoneal dissections.

   You have read the description of the technique and seen a lot of videos, maybe read my book.

   You have been to hands on trainings at the operation room and you have seen experienced colleagues perform LSCP.

   You have selected a simple case: first operation for POP, no previous history of pathologies inducing heavy peritoneal adhesions, the patient is skinny, she has no uterus or a normal sized one.

   You have reserved enough time in your schedule to be out of hurry.

   You did speak with your favorite anesthesiologist who is a very patient person and he knows that this is your first LSCP and that it will take some time. My first LSCP in 1993 took us 4 hours.

   You have all the instruments necessary to LSCP: something to present the cul de sacs, eventually something to suspend the annexes or the bowel, your favorite energy (I prefer harmonic scalpel for that operation), a good aspiration device, one or two good needle holders and eventually a knot pusher.

2. Start the dissection. You may encounter some problems. Let's detail them and try to find a simple solution.

   (a) **Dissection of the promontory is difficult**. You can see the promontory through the peritoneum but you can't free it. This is due to the fact that there are two layers of tissue above the promontory. One is the peritoneum; the other is a sub-peritoneal fascia. When you raise the peritoneum with the grip forceps in the left hand in order to bring it far away from the vessels, sometimes the fascia detaches and remains on the promontory. And when you incise the peritoneum, the fascia remains intact and you see no dissection plan leading to the para-rectal space and you don't visualize a free promontory. This is even more frequent in obese patients when fat is spread in between the layers. The solution is to grasp the fascia in front of the promontory and to incise it. Suddenly, you will see CO_2 pass through the incision, the promontory appears and the para-rectal space can be seen, looking like a soft white felting or a dense spider web.

   (b) **You have dissected the promontory and the iliac vein is covering it completely.** This is not frequent but justifies starting the dissection at the level of the promontory. You have two solutions: either you plan to suture the mesh to the prevertebral ligament at a lower level in the sacral concavity, below the vessels or you abandon LSCP for an alternative technique. If this is your first LSCP, I suggest you choose the second solution. It is never good to start with sophisticated and atypical procedures. Suturing at this level is more difficult and more risky because the ligament is frequently hard to pass with the needle and medial veins may exist and visibility is limited in the sacral concavity. You can move to open SCP or to vaginal repair of POP (see Chap. 12). Nevertheless, if you move to open LCP, I suggest you try to dissect laparoscopically the recto-vaginal and vesico-vaginal spaces to improve your skill. If you decide to continue the LSCP, be aware that using staplers or fasteners at the level of the sacral concavity is not very resistant and a suture should be preferred.

(c) **You have started the dissection of the recto-vaginal space but you are afraid of injuring the rectum and you didn't reach the levator muscles yet**. This is a frequent issue in the early experience, especially in case of big rectocele. The solution is easy: if you feel insecure after having pushed your recto-vaginal dissection as far as you think it is reasonable for you to do, after having checked if the cul de sac presenter is in the right position and decided that moving it doesn't improve your chances of going lower, stop the dissection and fix the posterior mesh directly to the vaginal wall with 2 sutures or 2 endohernia 4.8 mm staples or equivalents. Finish LSCP as in the manual and then raise the patient's legs and inspect the vagina. If there is a remnant low rectocele, fix it vaginally with a myorraphy or a fascial repair. This little problem may happen once or twice during the 10 first LSCP you will perform until you master completely this dissection. It should never be a reason to abandon LSCP.

(d) **The anterior dissection is tough due to a cesarean section scar**. Fibrosis around the Cesarean section (CS) scar is located in front of the cervix and is likely to extend 1 cm downwards to the vaginal cul de sac. It's just at the place you start your dissection and there's a big risk of bleeding if you enter the vaginal wall that is very well irrigated or to injury the bladder if you stay away from the vagina. What you can do is first to use the cul de sac presenter to visualize exactly where the vaginal wall is located. This may be enough to find the right dissection plane. If not, you should dissect more laterally, not too much because the ureters are crossing the parameters 1 cm laterally from the cervix. The adhesions to the CS scar are usually very medial and you can find the free vagina laterally. Then you follow it and you'll reach the medial part of the vagina below the adhesions to the scar. It makes it easy to cut the fibrous part and complete the dissection. You can make sure you didn't injury the bladder by looking at the urine bag: in case of injury, the bag is inflated. In this case, make a blue dye test to find the hole in the bladder and suture it according to your habits. We're used to suture it with Vicryl 00 in one layer. Insertion the anterior mesh in case of bladder injury is not contra indicated but you should leave the Foley catheter in place for at least 3–5 days according to the size of the defect.

(e) **A rectal injury occurs**. The rectum has to be sutured. According to your qualification and to the medico legal regulations in your place, you do it yourself or you call a colorectal surgeon. The suture may be done laparoscopically and if the defect is small, colostomy or ileostomy is not required systematically. But the POP repair should be cancelled: no synthetic mesh should be inserted on an injured rectum. The risk is to infect the mesh possibly leading to a spondylodiscitis.

Tricks and Tips: How to Make a Long Story Short?

8

LSCP is known as an operation that takes time! If we look at literature, abdominal open sacrocolpopexy takes about 3–4 h [1], LSCP 25 min to one hour more [2, 3] and robotic SCP (RSCP) again 40 min to 1 h more [4, 5] bringing it to over 4–5 h average in well trained hands. At least, we suppose they are well trained, because they publish. So we're afraid to guess how long it may take when a beginner performs it!

The team of Michel Cosson in Lille [6] has assessed the learning curve and found out that operative time for LSCP drops from 251 min average in beginners to 178 min after completed learning curve. How long is the learning curve? In RSCP, operation time drops from 5.3 to 3.6 h and plateaus after the 60 first procedures [7]. Amazingly, learning curve of LSCP seems to be shorter: operation time decreases from 196 to 162 min after 15 procedures for Mustafa [8] and after 18–24 procedures for Wattiez [9]. This may be explained by the fact that LSCP is performed by experienced surgeons, trained to highly advanced laparoscopy and maybe RSCP publications reflect the first experience of the surgeons with the robot. Thus, the learning curve is double: half to learn to use the robot and half to learn the technique of RSCP.

My personal experience is different. My learning curve was longer: it took me about 50 procedures to plateau my operative time which dropped from 4 h to 80 min average. We published results of the 44 first patients with an average operative time of 2 h 10 [10]. But I had nobody to teach me because in the early 90s, Wattiez, Cosson and me, we were the 3 first gynecologists to start with this procedure. Video facilities were poor. Instruments were poor. And the technique was not standardized.

In this chapter, I would like to share with you the tips and tricks I have developed during my surgical experience of the last 16 years to simplify and to make this procedure quicker.

© Springer International Publishing AG 2017
P. von Theobald, *Laparoscopic Sacrocolpopexy for Beginners*,
DOI 10.1007/978-3-319-57636-7_8

1. Avoid suturing when possible
   (a) EndoHernia stapler (Covidien): This endoscopic stapler has been designed
       in the late 90s to attach hernia meshes during laparoscopic repair. The stapler
       needs a 12 mm trocar. The 4.8 mm staples are designed for soft tissue like
       peritoneum, fascia, vaginal wall or even rectal wall. These staples allow fixa-
       tion of the mesh to the levator ani muscles, to the vaginal wall and to close
       easily and very quickly the peritoneal incisions. The depth of penetration is
       calibrated and constant of 2 mm; it's safe for fixation to structures like the
       vaginal wall that has a 5 mm thick wall. The 4.0 mm staples are for tough
       tissue like promontory or Cooper ligaments. The depth of 1.5 mm is secure
       at the promontory, as the thickness of the prevertebral ligament has been
       proven to be 1.4–2.3 mm [11]. I spare at least 30 min of operative time using
       this device.

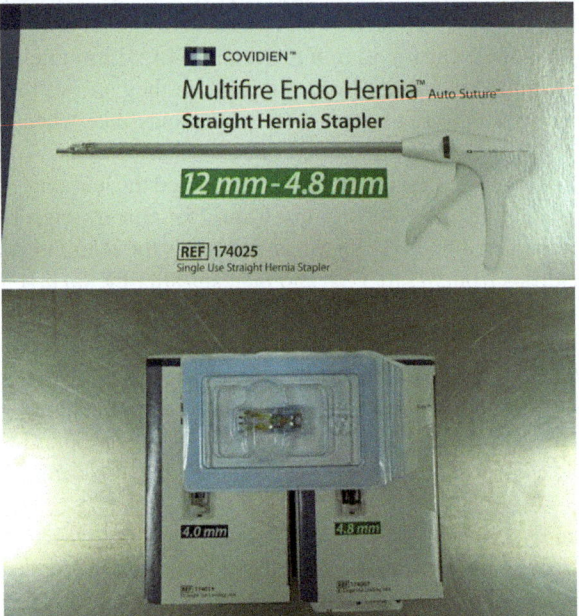

Picture: EndoHernia stapler and the additional cartridges of staples: 4.8 mm for soft
tissue and 4.0 mm for the promontory

   (b) Securestrap (Ethicon): it's an absorbable staple with which you can fix the
       mesh to the levator ani muscles and to the promontory. Its advantage is to be
       a 5 mm device and to deliver an absorbable implant. But you cannot fix the
       mesh to the vagina because the depth of penetration is too long and you
       cannot close the peritoneum with it. But you'll save at least 20 min of
       operative time.

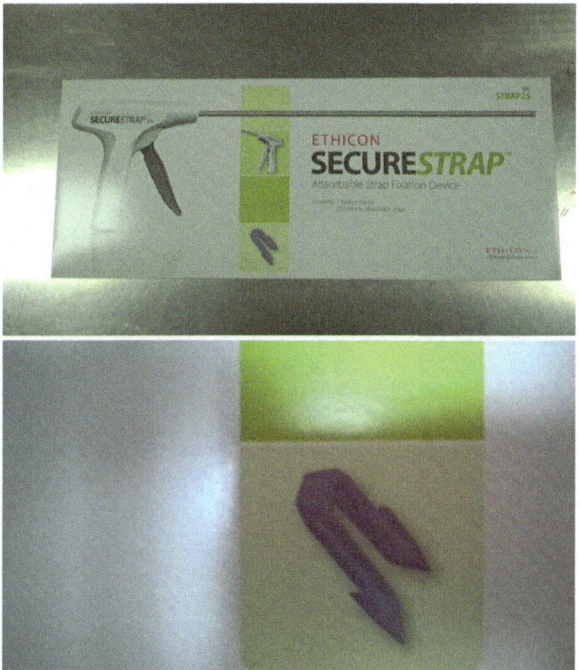

Picture: The SecureStrap stapler. The staples are slowly absorbable

(c) EndoFast Reliant SCP (Allium-medical): this is a very new device that can
be used to fix very easily the mesh to the promontory, to the elevator muscles and to the vagina because of its very limited and calibrated depth of
penetration. The device is very effective due to the "spider fastener" (see
picture) the anchors the mesh in a very reliable way with its six bended
arms. It passes through a 5 mm trocar. But it doesn't help you to close the
peritoneum.

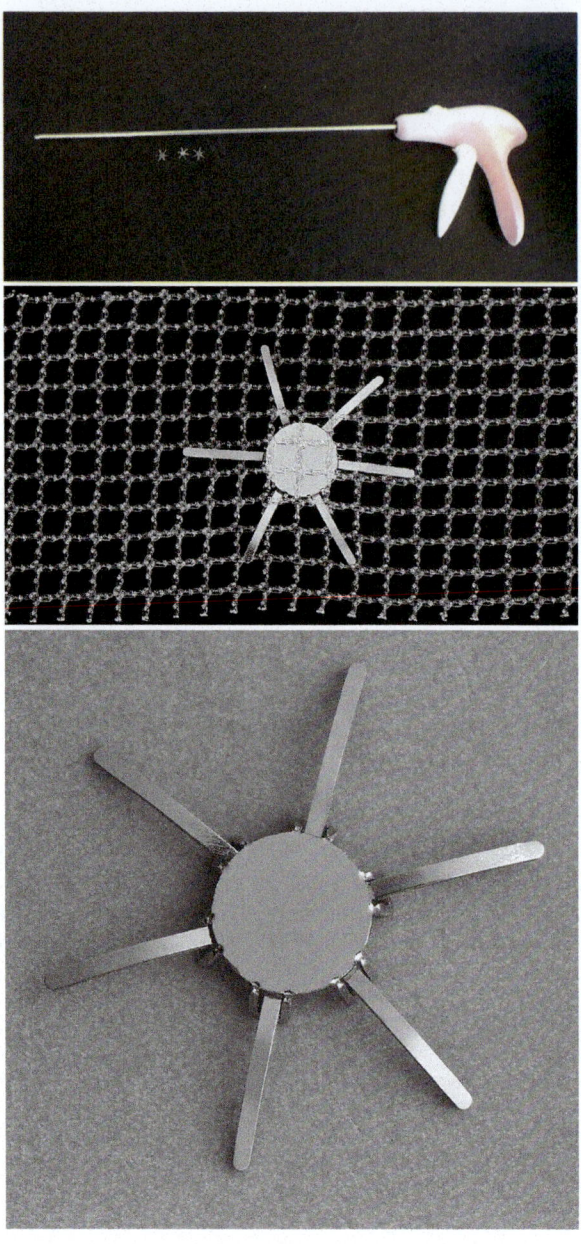

Pictures: The EndoFast Reliant SCP stapler can be used for promontory and elevator muscles

(d) Glue: Interesting idea published by two French teams [12, 13]. The first teams claimed a reduction of operative time and the second found no difference. The glue was used to fix the anterior and posterior meshes to the levator ani muscles and to the vaginal wall only. Not to the promontory and both teams sutured the meshes to the uterine isthmus or to the vaginal vault. Thus, in fact, using glue was more or less an additional step and time sparing could only be due to inserting less sutures. The team that spared time skipped the levator and vagina sutures. The other team did not. None tried to close the peritoneum also with glue, which would be a great step ahead, I think, if it works.

(e) Tacker: I don't recommend using the metallic tacker to fix the mesh to the promontory nor to the vagina. This device is very efficient but several case reports of migration into the bladder and spondylodiscitis have been published. It seems that this device is penetrating too deep into the structures, passing through the pre-vertebral ligament into the discus [11]. Thus, in case of infection, it may affect the vertebral disc immediately. If used on the vaginal wall, as it is a metallic smooth device, it may migrate into bladder or bowel.

2. Use T-Lift device to expose the Douglas pouch: when the patient is obese or when the sigmoid colon is very long and makes it difficult to expose the dissection area, T-Lift is a very useful device. Push the needle under view control through the sigmoid meso or through a fatty appendix, slide the T-shaped plastic strip through the needle and suspend the organ to the abdominal wall. You can also suspend the ovaries or the uterine body. T-Lift is a cheap device, easy to use and helping greatly to spare operative time.

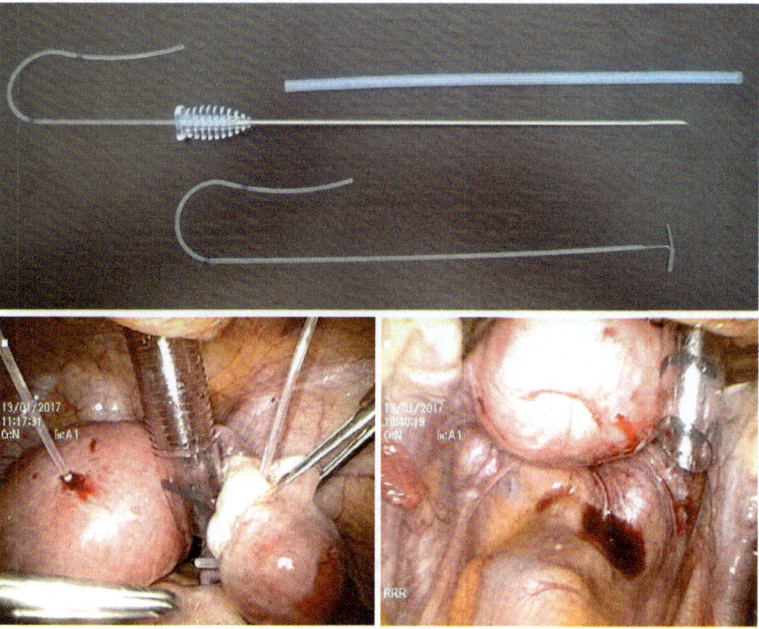

3. Suture peritoneum with auto locking sutures: These sutures are available since 2010. We use VLock 2/0 absorbable sutures for vaginal closure after hysterectomy, for bladder closure in case of injury and for closure of the peritoneum. It saves a lot of time because your assistant doesn't need to hold the continuous suture and can help you in presenting the tissue that has to be sutured.

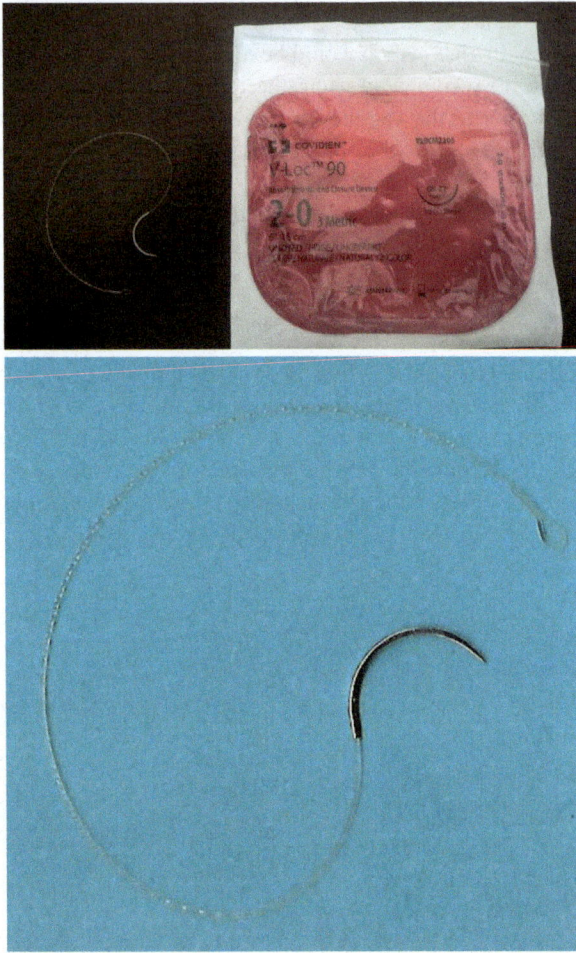

4. Avoid useless hysterectomy as described on Chap. 5. A very recent meta-analysis by Maher [14] shows that there's no evidence to support the need of hysterectomy to improve results. And if you follow the technique described in this book, laparaoscopic sacro-hystero-colpopexy takes much less time than laparoscopic sacrocolpopexy with supracervical hysterectomy. Of course, this is indicated only in women without medical need for hysterectomy.

5. Use a two armed anterior mesh to avoid sutures to the vagina. Using the two armed mesh allows a very quick anchoring of the anterior and posterior mesh to the uterine isthmus without any suture. Fenestration of the broad ligament is an easy, quick and blunt procedure. The anterior sheet of the ligament is already incised after vesico-vaginal dissection. You grasp the end of the mesh arm with a laparoscopic forceps and rub it softly through the connective tissue, laterally from the uterine vessels and branches, until you can see by transparence the forceps through the posterior sheet. The either you incise it or you just push firmly the forceps holding the mesh through the sheet. You perform the same procedure on the opposite and you can knot the two arms together behind the cervix and behind the posterior mesh. This saves at least 20 min of time.

6. Keep peritoneal incision medial to the right utero-sacral ligament (see picture). This is more than a tip. When you have opened the peritoneum at the level of the promontory, you continue the dissection down to the Douglas pouch and the recto-vaginal plane. Many surgeons are afraid of having a rectal injury and stay far away from this organ, making a very lateral dissection. The risk of being too far from the right side of the rectum is to become lateral to the right uterosacral ligament. Thus you may cross the way of the right ureter and injury it. You will also leave the pararectal space that is fatty but avascular, allowing mainly blunt dissection to arrive in the retroperitoneal space where you'll find the hypo gastric vessels. It is very important to check the position of the uterosacral ligament by pulling firmly on the rectum when you make the dissection between promontory and Douglas pouch to stay secure and to find the para rectal space.

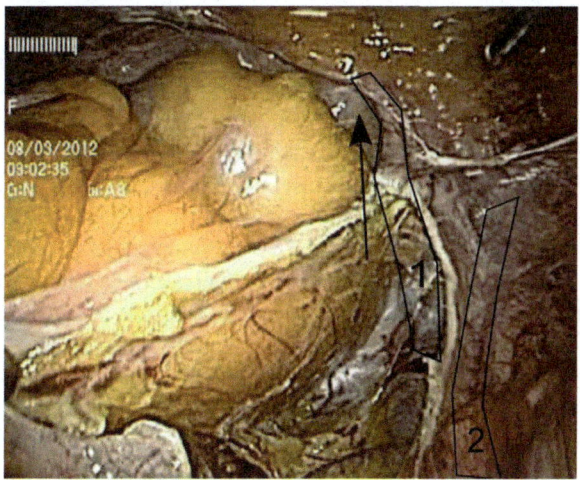

Picture: The peritoneal incision, parallel to the rectum, must stay medial to the right utero sacral ligament (*1*) in order to stay far away from the right ureter (*2*)

7. Start dissection at posterior vaginal wall in case of vault prolapse: very frequently after total hysterectomy, the bladder overlaps the vaginal scar (picture). The risk of bladder injury is big if you try to dissect at first the anterior vaginal wall. Furthermore, the dissection plane is very fibrous at the site of the vaginal scar which is on the anterior wall. The trick is to open the peritoneum at the basis of the posterior wall and to "unwrap" progressively the vault and then the lateral parts of the anterior wall and to finish with the central dissection of the scar (picture?). Don't remove the dissected peritoneum; keep it attached to the bladder and use it in the end to facilitate the peritonization. This technique will save time because you go from the easy part of the dissection to the tough one and it will also save time in reducing the risk of bladder injury.

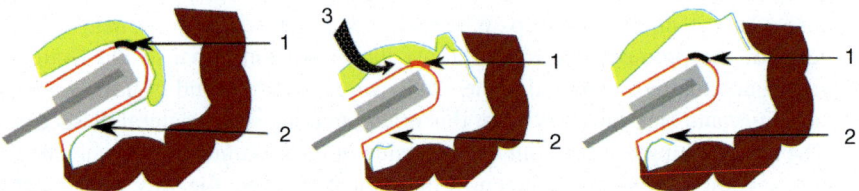

Picture: dissection of the vaginal vault (*1* vaginal hysterectomy scar, *2* place to start the dissection, *3* lateral dissection of the bladder before freeing the scar)

8. Use harmonic energy. There is no best energy. Any energy has pros and cons. The best energy is certainly the one you're used to and that you master. It may be monopolar, bipolar current, harmonic energy or plasmajet. The fact is that the dissection planes you will encounter in LSCP are mainly avascular. The will normally be no big vessel to seal. Main bleeding comes from the sub peritoneal micro-vascularization and from the fatty tissue of the para rectal space, especially in obese women. Any of these energies may fix it. So why do we recommend harmonic? First, we avoid monopolar because of thermal spread. Bipolar energy is excellent will small risk of lateral tissue burns but bipolar devices don't cut. That means that you'll have to use another instrument, a scissor, to cut the cauterized tissue. At each cauterization you'll have to change the instrument and, as you progress 5 per 5 mm, to dissect 10 cm will require 20 changes of instruments. This is a waste of time. Harmonic scalpel is a multifunctional tool that can dissect, grasp, cauterize and cut the tissue. Final result: no change of instrument and at least 20 min less operative time in the end.

9. Use a tunneler: If a tunneler is available, you will spare a lot of time because you just dissect the promontory and the rectovaginal space down to the elevators. You don't open the peritoneum along the right side of the rectum and thus, you will not be obliged to close it afterwards. The Neymeyer tunneler (see pictures below), sold by SERAG WIESSNER is easy to use. Just make sure you always stay medial to the right utero sacral ligament to avoid problems with the right ureter.

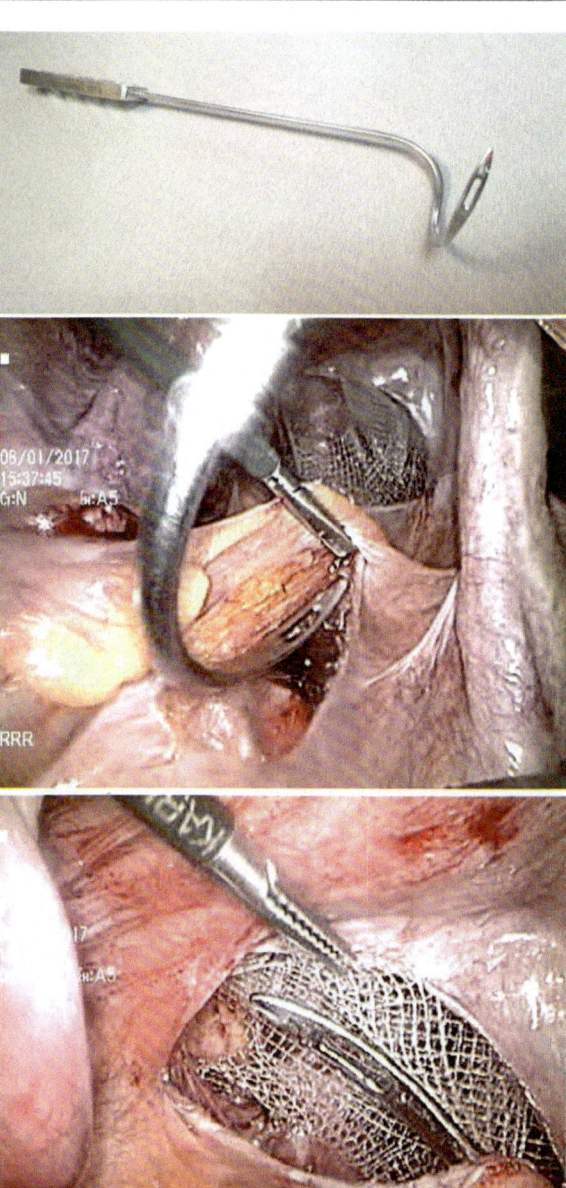

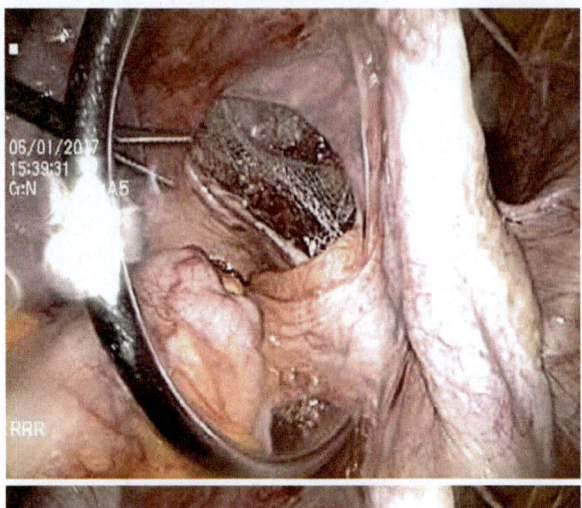

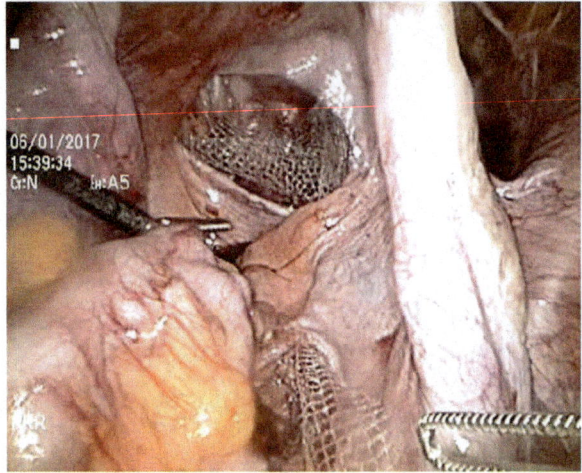

References

1. Hsiao KC, Latchamsetty K, Govier FE, Kozlowski P, Kobashi KC. Comparison of laparoscopic and abdominal sacrocolpopexy for the treatment of vaginal vault prolapse. J Endourol. 2007 Aug;21(8):926–30.
2. Campbell P, Cloney L, Jha S. Abdominal versus laparoscopic Sacrocolpopexy: a systematic review and meta-analysis. Obstet Gynecol Surv. 2016 Aug;71(7):435–42.
3. De Gouveia De Sa M, Claydon LS, Whitlow B, Dolcet Artahona MA. Laparoscopic versus open sacrocolpopexy for treatment of prolapse of the apical segment of the vagina: a systematic review and meta-analysis. Int Urogynecol J. 2016 Jan;27(1):3–17.
4. Callewaert G, Bosteels J, Housmans S, Verguts J, Van Cleynenbreugel B, Van der Aa F, De Ridder D, Vergote I, Deprest J. Laparoscopic versus robotic-assisted sacrocolpopexy for pelvic organ prolapse: a systematic review. Gynecol Surg. 2016;13:115–23.

5. Pan K, Zhang Y, Wang Y, Wang Y, Xu H. A systematic review and meta-analysis of conventional laparoscopic sacrocolpopexy versus robot-assisted laparoscopic sacrocolpopexy. Int J Gynaecol Obstet. 2016 Mar;132(3):284–91.
6. Vandendriessche D, Giraudet G, Lucot JP, Behal H, Cosson M. Impact of laparoscopic sacrocolpopexy learning curve on operative time, perioperative complications and short term results. Eur J Obstet Gynecol Reprod Biol. 2015 Aug;191:84–9.
7. Linder BJ, Anand M, Weaver AL, Woelk JL, Klingele CJ, Trabuco EC, Occhino JA, Gebhart JB. Assessing the learning curve of robotic sacrocolpopexy. Int Urogynecol J. 2016 Feb;27(2):239–46.
8. Mustafa S, Amit A, Filmar S, Deutsch M, Netzer I, Itskovitz-Eldor J, Lowenstein L. Implementation of laparoscopic sacrocolpopexy: establishment of a learning curve and short-term outcomes. Arch Gynecol Obstet. 2012 Oct;286(4):983–8.
9. Akladios CY, Dautun D, Saussine C, Baldauf JJ, Mathelin C, Wattiez A. Laparoscopic sacrocolpopexy for female genital organ prolapse: establishment of a learning curve. Eur J Obstet Gynecol Reprod Biol. 2010 Apr;149(2):218–21.
10. Cheret A, Von Theobald P, Lucas J, Dreyfus M, Herlicoviez M. Laparoscopic promontofixation feasibility study in 44 patients. J Gynecol Obstet Biol Reprod. 2001 Apr;30(2):139–43.
11. Estrade JP, Gurriet B, Franquebalme JP, Chinchole JM, Glowaczower E, Ferry C, Crochet P, Agostini A. Laparoscopic sacrocolpopexy with a vaginal prosthetic adhesive. Gynecol Obstet Fertil. 2015 Jun;43(6):419–23.
12. Graham E, Akl A, Brubaker L, Dhaher Y, Fitzgerald C, Mueller ER. Investigation of sacral needle depth in minimally invasive Sacrocolpopexy. Female Pelvic Med Reconstr Surg. 2016 Jul–Aug;22(4):214–8.
13. Willecocq C, Pizzoferrato AC, Fauconnier A, Bader G. Use of glue in laparoscopic sacrocolpopexy. A comparative study about 32 cases. Gynecol Obstet Fertil. 2014 Dec;42(12):822–6.
14. Costantini E, Brubaker L, Cervigni M, Matthews CA, O'Reilly BA, Rizk D, Giannitsas K, Maher CF. Sacrocolpopexy for pelvic organ prolapse: evidence-based review and recommendations. Eur J Obstet Gynecol Reprod Biol. 2016 Aug 3;205:60–5.

Short and Long Term Results: What Can You Expect Following LSCP?

We have published [1] a retrospective monocentric single operator series of all laparoscopic sacrocolpopexies performed for genital prolapse, according to the double mesh technique described in this book at the unit of Gynecology of the University Hospital of Caen between January 1993 and December 2002. We excluded patients who had laparoscopic mesh suspension for Masters and Allen Syndrome [2] as well as those who had a conversion to laparotomy for any reason. Patients were found through the French hospital discharge data base, the Programme of Medicalisation of Information System (PMSI) and all the hospital files as well as the operative and consultation reports were reviewed by two independent investigators.

The procedures have all been performed by me using the same surgical technique previously described for first 44 women [3, 4]. Laparoscopic Burch colposuspension [5] was almost systematically performed between 1993 and 2000. Later, TVT was used but only in case of objective stress urinary incontinence (SUI).

The study has been conducted in three steps. First step was the analysis of the medical files in order to gather pre, per and post operative data like BMI, previous history, staging of the POP according to the *International Continence Society (ICS): Pelvic Organ Prolapse Quantification POP-Q* [6], SUI, surgical report, associated procedures (hysterectomy, ovariectomy, etc.), complications. Second step was an observational descriptive evaluation. All the patients were directly contacted by phone first (to get their agreement participate, confirmed later by signature) and by mail (questionnaire). Quality of life (QoL) has been evaluated with the French validated short version of Pelvic Floor Distress Inventory 20 (PDFI 20) with the three sub groups of questions: Urinary Distress Inventory (UDI 6), Colo-Rectal and Anal Distress Inventory (CRADI 8) and Pelvic Organ Prolaps Distress Inventory (POPDI 6). Pelvic Floor Impact Questionnaire (PFIQ 7) has also been completed. This questionnaire has also three sub groups: Urinary Impact Questionnaire (UIQ 7), Colo-Rectal and Anal Impact Questionnaire (CRAIQ 7) et Pelvic Organ Prolaps Impact Questionnaire (POPIQ 7) [7, 8]. Last step was a clinical assessment of the anatomy. This examination, performed by an independent

© Springer International Publishing AG 2017
P. von Theobald, *Laparoscopic Sacrocolpopexy for Beginners*,
DOI 10.1007/978-3-319-57636-7_9

gynecologist (EM), was standardized to assess the anatomical defects according to ICS POP-Q. For the purpose of statistical data analysis, qualitative variables were described as frequency and percentages and quantitative ones as mean (ranges). To analyse risk factors for relapse we used chi-squares (or Fisher exact test) or t-test (or Mann-Whitney tests), as appropriate. The level of significance was set to 0.05 for these main analyses (bi sided tests). Analyses were carried out at the "Unité de Biostatistique et Recherche Clinique" (Caen University Hospital) using SPPS software vs 19.

9.1　Our Results

Out of the 104 women who had a LSCP between 1993 and 2002, six patients have deceased (5.8%) and 18 (17.3%) were impossible to contact despite repeated attempts. Eighty women were contacted and all of them accepted to participate to the study and to answer the questionnaires. Fifty-one patients accepted to meet the gynecologist for a clinical assessment (Fig. 9.1).

Average follow up was 13.6 years (range 11–20 years). Main characteristics of the population are described in Table 9.1. Preoperatively, 55% of patients showed

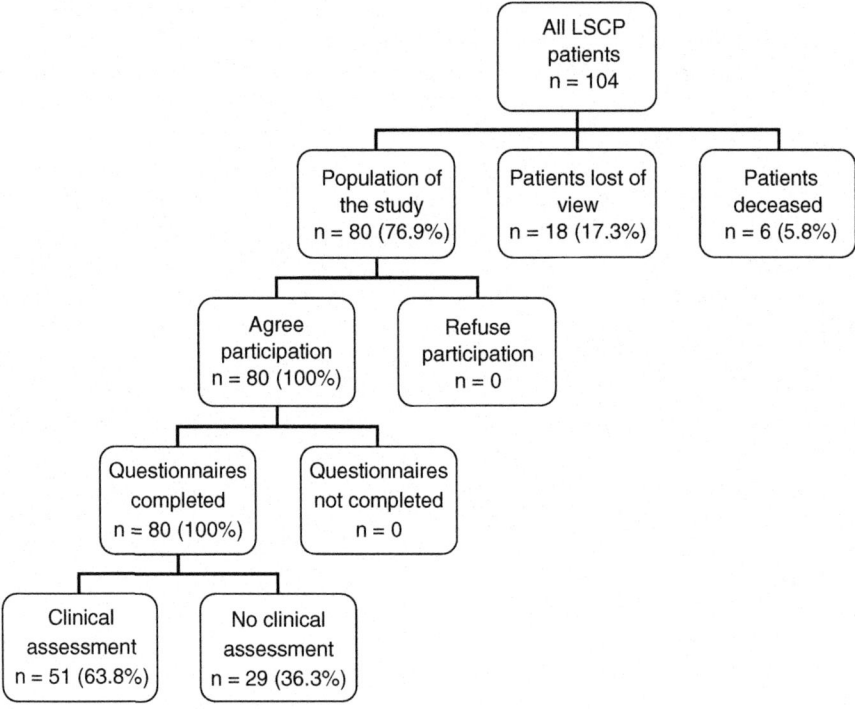

Fig. 9.1 Population of the study

Table 9.1 Clinical characteristics of the population of the study

Age at LSCP	54.4 [35–77]
Age at study	69.1 [46–91]
Body mass index (kg/m^2)	23.8 [18.4–36.3]
Parity	2.9 [1–7]
Ménopausal n (%)	52 (65%)
Previous hysterectomy n (%) Abdominal Vaginal	19 (23.8%) 11 (13.8%) 8 (10%)
Previous POP repair n (%) Abdominal Vaginal	16 (20%) 3 (3.8%) 13 (16.3%)
Previous SUI repair n (%)	9 (11.3%)
Pre operative symptoms n (%)	
Pelvic heaviness Urinary symptoms Bowel symptoms	79 (98.8%) 38 (47.5%) 6 (7.5%)

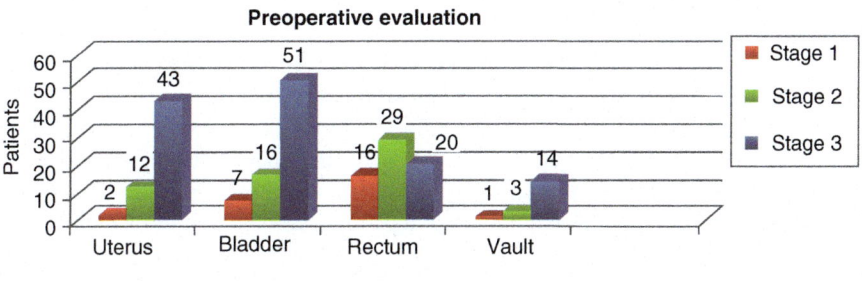

Fig. 9.2 Preoperative clinical evaluation (POP-Q)

a prolapse of the three compartments (n = 44) and 45% of complained of SUI (n = 36). Preoperative characteristics are on Fig. 9.2. Average operation duration, including associated procedures, was 130 min (60–220). Subtotal hysterectomy was performed in 3 patients (3.8%) and SUI repair in 50 patients (62.5%). Eight preoperative complications (10%) occurred: six bladder injuries and two vaginal injuries. Short term results have been published in 2001 for the 44 first patient of this series [10].

9.1.1   Long Term Anatomic Results

After average follow up of 13.6 years (11–20), 20 women have been re operated for recurrence (25%). In 19 of these, only one compartment recurred. In 11 patients (55% of recurrences), it appeared to be a cystocele, in 7 patients (35%) a

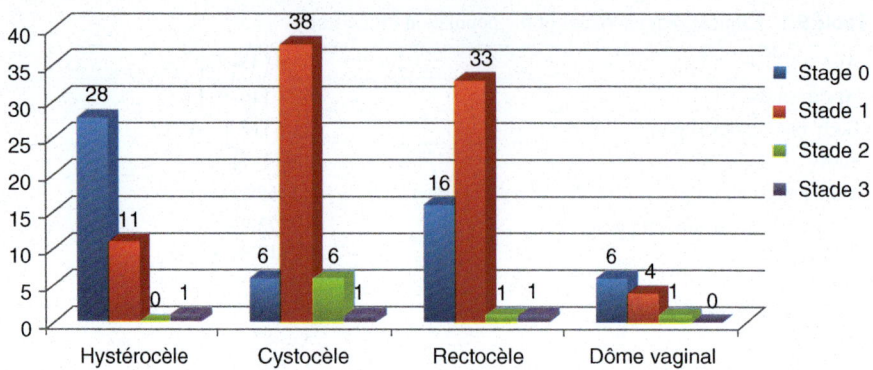

Fig. 9.3 Long term follow up anatomical results (POP-Q)

rectocele and in 2 patients (10%) a uterine prolapse. Recurrence happened after 5.9 years for cystocele, 7.4 years for rectocele and 7.3 tears for vault or uterine descent. POP-Q staging of the 51 patients that could be examined clinically is on Figs. 9.2 and 9.3. Eleven women (21.5%) had a recurrence (POP-Q = 2 or more). In seven women (63.6%), it was a cystocele. Recurrence was asymptomatic in eight women (72.7%). Six of the patients with recurrence have had a second operation during the follow up period and four of them presented a recurrence on the compartment that has been reoperated (always cystocele). Among the 80 women of our study, 15 (18.8%) had a SUI repair during the follow up period after 6.4 years average. The SUI repair was associated with POP repair in five women (33.3%). At the time of the evaluation, five patients complained of de novo SUI.

9.1.2   Risk Factors for Recurrence

We were looking for correlations between previous history, BMI, initial POP-Q stage and recurrence. The only significant correlation was with the presence of a large cystocele at the beginning (Tables 9.2 and 9.3).

9.1.3   Long Term Functional Results

Functional results are described on Table 9.4 and evolution of symptoms and QoL on Table 9.5. Urinary symptoms were mainly urinary incontinence and/or bladder over activity. Recurrence happened after 8.9 years average. In 66.7% of women (n = 10), no recurrence of POP was associated. After analyzing the QoL questionnaires, 92.5% of patients had no more urinary symptom (UDI-7 score of 20/100) and 93.8% had no impairment of QoL (UDI score 10.8/100). Pelvic symptoms were mainly heaviness and discomfort. Recurrence happened after 8.9 years average.

Table 9.2 Risk factors for recurrence

	n/N	(%)	p
Multiparity			
yes	20/76	26.3%	*0.568*
no	0/4	0%	
Menopausal			
yes	14/52	26.9%	*0.852*
No	6/28	21.4%	
Previous hysterectomy			
yes	4/19	21.1%	*1000*
No	16/61	26.2%	
Previous POP repair			
yes	1/15	6.7%	*0.331*
No	19/65	29.2%	
Uterie descent stage 3			
yes	13/43	30.2%	*0.517*
No	3/16	18.8%	
Cystocele stage 3			
yes	17/51	33.3%	**0.049**
No	3/29	10.3%	
Rectocele stage 3			
yes	16/60	26.7%	*0.883*
No	4/20	20%	
Vault prolapse stage 3			
yes	4/14	28.6%	*1000*
no	1/5	20%	
Hysterectomy during LSCP			
yes	0/3	0%	*0.563*
No	20/77	25.9%	

Table 9.3 BMI and recurrence

	N	average	Standard deviation	p Mann-Whitney
BMI ≥ 25				
yes	20	24	3.2	0.225
No	80	23.4	3.2	

At the time of our study, 96.3% of women presented no symptom (POPDI-6 score 14/100) and 95% had no impairment of QoL (POPQI-7 Score 7.5/100). Rectal symptoms were mainly constipation and/or obstructed defecation and recurrence happened after 6.8 years average (1–11 years). In 80% of women, constipation was associated with POP recurrence. 86.3% of patients didn't complain of bowel symptoms (CRADI-8 score 20.2/100) and 93.1% had no impairment of QoL (CRAIQ-7 score 12/100).

Table 9.4 Long term functional results

	Urinary symptoms	Pelvic symptoms	Defecation <3 per week
Patients symptomatic before surgery			
n (%)	38 (47.5%)	79 (98.8%)	6 (7.5%)
Patients symptomatic after follow up			
n (%)	15 (18.8%)	6 (7.5%)	10 (12.5%)
Unchanged	28 (35%)	6 (7.5%)	6 (7.5%)
Worse	10 (12.5%)	0	2 (2.5%)
De novo	5 (6.3%)	0	2 (2.5%)

Table 9.5 Long term evaluation of QoL

	Evaluation of POP symptoms n (%)	Evaluation of QoL n (%)
Improved	64 (80%)	74 (92.5%)
Unchanged	15 (18.8%)	5 (6.3%)
Worse	1 (1.3%)	1 (1.3%)

9.1.4   Long Term Dyspareunia

Twenty-seven patients were still sexually active at the time of the study (33.7%) and five complained of de novo dyspareunia. Among the 42 patients that were not sexually active, none complained of de novo dyspareunia after the LSCP until the end of their sexual life.

9.1.5   Long Term Complication Rate

Global rate of long term complications is 11.3% (9 patients) including 5 vaginal mesh erosion, exposition or rejection occurring after 7.2 years (3–12), 4 incisional hernias occurring after 4.8 years (1–10) in women with BMI > 25 for 3 of them.

9.2   Discussion

There are few data in literature about long term results of LSCP [9]. A review is on Table 9.6. Higgs et al. reported retrospective results after a median of 66 months in 103 women with vault prolapse [10]. Surgical technique was heterogeneous in this series; some women had a double approach (vaginal and laparoscopic) for mesh insertion with a high vaginal erosion rate. Some had a single mesh sutured to the vault and the promontory with high anterior and posterior compartment recurrence. Some had laparoscopic insertion of a long posterior mesh and sometimes an additional anterior mesh. Granese et al. [11] reported a series with 43 months of follow up in 138 women with vault prolapse. Technique was close to ours. No validated QoL were used. Bowel symptoms like constipation and obstructed defecation increased during follow up from 7% to 13% and from 1.5% to 5.8% respectively.

Table 9.6 Review of literature

		Higgs	Granese	Sergent	Sarlos	Rivoire	Bui	Our series
Study type		Retrospective	Prospective	Prospective	Prospective	Retrospective	Prospective	Retrospective
Patients		103	138	116	85	131	84	80
Prolapse		Vault	Vault	All	All	All	All	All
Age at study		?	67 (58–76)	52.2 (30–70)	?	60.4 +/– 9.5	54 (30–75)	69.1 (46–91)
Clinical examination		66	?	116	68	108	84	51
QoL questionnaire		103	?	116	85	131	84	80
Follow up (months)		66 (37–124)	43 (6–96)	34.2 (+/–20.5)	60	33.7 +/– 17.4	30.7 (7–102)	164 (132–240)
Long term complications	Vaginal erosions (%)	9.0%	0.70%	3.40%	0%	5%	1.20%	6.2%
	Spondylodis-citis (n)	0	0	1	0	1	1	0
	Other	0	0	1 recto vaginal fistula	2 bladder erosion	1 vesico vaginal fistula	1 chronic pain	4 incision hernias
Anatomic recurrence	Anterior	22.70%	11.60%	12.2%	8.8%	17.5%	12.5%	21.5%
	Apical	4.0%	5%	2.6%	1.5%	13.7%	1.0%	3.9%
	Posterior	28.0%	12.30%	1.7%	5.9%	8.3%	9.5%	3.9%
Reoperation rate for POP		16.0%	20.20%	?	5.8%	5.0%	?	25.0%

(continued)

Table 9.6 (continued)

		Higgs	Granese	Sergent	Sarlos	Rivoire	Bui	Our series
Subjective cure	Global	79.0%	83.30%	?	95.3%	98.0%	81%	93.8%
	De novo constipation/obstructed defecation	?	18.80%	1.70%	4.7%	14.0%	13%	2.5%
	De novo SUI	?	5%	5%	37.6%	?	21.40%	6.3%
	De novo dyspareunia (among sexually active)	46.0%	3%	1%	24.0%	0.0%	15.70%	18.5%
	Sexually active	58.2%	?	73%	48.0%	61.0%	83.30%	33.7%
Reoperation rate for SUI		11.0%	?	?	18.8%	5.0%	?	18.8%

Sergent et al. [12] published a prospective observational study of 116 women with POP, using the same QoL questionnaires as in our series and with a mean follow up of 34.2 months. Fifty-six subtotal hysterectomies (48.2%) and 29 SUI (25%) repairs were performed concurrently (vs 3.8% and 62.5% in our series). QoL questionnaires (PFDI, PFDIQ, and PPISQ-12) showed all significant improvement without impairment of bowel symptoms as in our series, maybe because of the younger age of the patients at the end of the follow up. The highest rate of anatomical failures was observed on anterior compartment. Sarlos et al. [13] published a prospective study of 85 women with POP and 60 months of follow. Supracervical hysterectomy, if uterine prolapse present, was systematic in this series. Most of recurrences occurred on the anterior compartment and within 12 months after initial surgery. Constipation rate increases from 1% one year after surgery to 4.7% at 5 years. Bui et al. [14] presented a prospective series of 84 women with 30.7 months of follow up. Eighty-three women had hysterectomy among the 92 still having their uterus. As in our series, anorectal scores (CRADI-8 and CRAIQ-7) showed impairment in time. The de novo dyspareunia rate is high contrasting with the improved PISQ-12 score. No explanation was provided. Rivoire et al. [15] published a retrospective series of 131 women with 33.7 months of follow up. Technique was similar to our series but almost all had supracervical hysterectomy at the time of the LSCP. No QoL score was used to evaluate subjective results but 14% of patients had de novo constipation after LSCP. Urinary symptoms were not detailed but 51% of women were incontinent before and 47% after procedure despite 86% associated SUI repairs, mainly Burch colposuspension as in our series.

Our series had an average follow up of 156 months and showed a high recurrence rate (25% reoperation, 21.5% at examination) happening after 5.9, 7.3 and 7.4 years for anterior, apical and posterior compartment respectively. SUI recurred after 8.9 years, pelvic symptoms after 8.9 years and rectal symptoms after 6.8 years average. Vaginal mesh erosion happened after 7.2 years average, later than after vaginal mesh insertion in literature: 41% after 24 months [16], but similar to the series of Higgs et al. with vaginal incision [10]. Our study demonstrates that recurrences and complication occur much later than the end of follow up of all the analyzed studies and thus, results and complication rates of LSCP appear to be optimistic and have to be revised.

If anatomic results are deteriorating in time, amazingly, QoL is not degraded; scores demonstrate no impairment of Qol in 92.8–95% of women which is consistent with the results of all other series having a shorter follow up except for Higgs [10], probably explained by the heterogeneity of the surgical techniques in his series. The difference between anatomic and functional outcomes underlines the usefulness of validated QoL questionnaires to indicate surgery and to evaluate results [7]. Improving function should be our first target.

Spondylodiscitis, occurred three times in the review (0.4%) and four other severe complications as recto and vesico vaginal fistula and mesh erosion into the bladder were reported. Incisional hernias were not reported in any series but ours. A recent publication [17] found an incidence of 3.5% in laparoscopic surgery after a follow up of 32.2 months. Obesity was a risk factor as in our series.

In all series (except for Granese [11] and Higgs [10] who did not systematically reinforce the recto vaginal fascia by a posterior mesh), anatomic recurrence occurs mainly on anterior compartment. We found that a preexisting large cystocele was a risk factor for recurrence. Unfortunately we didn't quote precisely the anatomic defects of the vesico vaginal fascia in our preoperative assessment. We think that defects like lateral detachment from the arcus tendineous or even low central defects cannot be repaired by an abdominal approach. LSCP can only reattach the fascia to the pericervical ring and reinforce the fascia at the upper half of the anterior vagina, above the level of the trigone. For women with a big cystocele, with lateral defect, vaginal approach with mesh might theoretically be the best solution. Unfortunately, no long term results nor specific comparative trial have been published to date, only series with 3 years follow up [18, 19]. A randomized French study is ongoing [20].

Anorectal function after LSCP seems to be impaired in most mid-term series [11, 13–15] as on long term in our series but impact on measured QoL is little. It may be due to pararectal or presacral dissection causing nerve lesions [15].

Our series describes the result of our first 104 LSCP, including our learning curve as in 4 of the 6 reviewed publications [10, 11, 14, 15]. According to David [21] LSCP learning in an experimented surgical team induces high operative time, but remains safe for patient and doesn't modify outcome. As reported in a previous publication about short term results in 44 women of the same series [3], operation time was 240 min in the very first patients an decreased to 155 minutes after 30 operations, as in most series [9].

Performing supracervical hysterectomy at the time of LSCP is the rule in literature [12–15]. This is a difference with our series; we systematically preserved the uterus unless there was a specific medical reason, like myoma or adenomyosis, to remove it (in three patients only). This fact, added to the length of the follow up, may have influenced the outcomes.

We acknowledge that our series has some potential sources of bias: it's a retrospective study and 23% of patients were lost of view. The numbers are too small to evaluate some risk factors for recurrence like BMI or hysterectomy or to rate rare complications like spondylodiscitis.

9.3   In Summary

Long term results of LSCP performed with the described double mesh technique are finally good according to satisfaction index and QoL questionnaires. But 25% of patients had to be re operated average 5–8 years after first procedure, mainly for recurrent cystocele. This means that the results published in most series with a follow up between 1 and 3 years are truly overoptimistic (Fig. 9.4).

Pre existing large cystocele is a risk factor for anterior compartment recurrence. In this case, vaginal repair with mesh should be discussed.

Long term complication rate is low but some complications may be severe. As complications occur after a long period, the complication rate is also

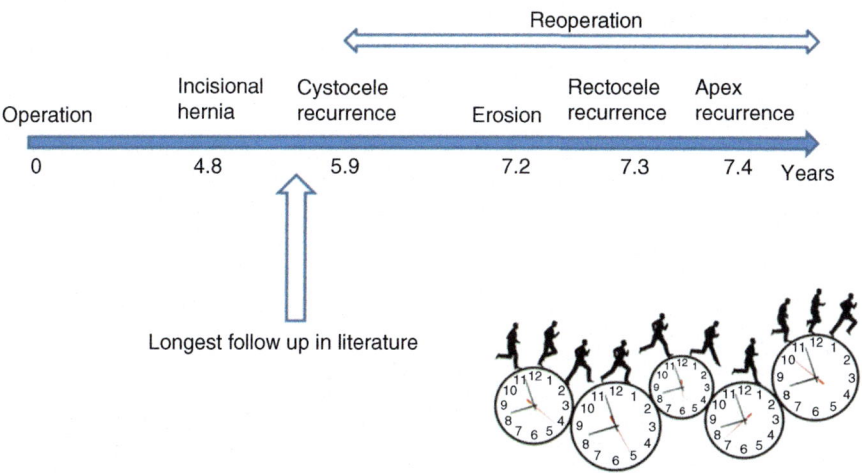

Fig. 9.4 Timeline for average occurrence of recurrences and complications

underestimated in literature. Some complications, like incisional hernia, are never mentioned in series despite a known incidence of more than 3.5% after 3 years.

References

1. Massou E, Chéret A, Marcus-Braun N, von Theobald P. Laparoscopic sacro(hystero)colpopexy: twenty years after. Women's Health & Gynecology. 2016 Apr 7. http://scientonline.org/open-access/laparoscopic-sacrohysterocolpopexy-twenty-years-after.pdf
2. von Theobald P, Barjot P, Levy G. Laparoscopic douglasectomy in the treatment of painful uterine retroversion. Surg Endosc. 1997;11(6):639–42.
3. Cheret A, Von Theobald P, Lucas J, Dreyfus M, Herlicoviez M. Laparoscopic promontofixation feasibility study in 44 patients. J Gynecol Obstet Biol Reprod. 2001 Apr;30(2):139–43.
4. von Theobald P. Laparoscopic promontofixation. J Chir. 2001 Dec;138(6):353–7.
5. von Theobald P, Barjot P, Liegeois P, Herlicoviez M, Levy G. Laparoscopic colpo-suspension by the Burch technique. Presse Med. 1994;23(28):1301–3.
6. Bump RC, Mattiasson A, Bø K, Brubaker LP, DeLancey JO, Klarskov P, Shull BL, Smith AR. The standardisation of terminology of female pelvic organ prolapse and pelvic floor dysfunction from the international continence society committee on standardisation of terminology, subcommittee on pelvic organ prolapse and pelvic floor dysfunction. Am J Obstet Gynecol. 1996;175:10–7.
7. de Tayrac R, Letouzey V. The use of quality of life scales in women with pelvic organ prolapse: gadget or real progress ? Gynecol Obstet Fertil. 2011;39(3):125–6.
8. de Tayrac R, Deval B, Fernandez H, Marès P. Mapi research institute. Development of a linguistically validated French version of two short-form, condition-specific quality of life questionnaires for women with pelvic floor disorders (PFDI-20 and PFIQ-7). J Gynecol Obstet Biol Reprod. 2007;36(8):738–48.
9. Ganatra AM, Rozet F, Sanchez-Salas R, Barret E, Galiano M, Cathelineau X, Vallancien G. The current status of laparoscopic sacrocolpopexy: a review. Eur Urol. 2009;55(5):1089–103.

10. Higgs PJ, Chua HL, Smith AR. Long-term review of laparoscopic sacrocolpopexy. Br J Obstet Gynaecol. 2005;112:1134–8.
11. Granese R, Candiani M, Perino A, Romano F, Cucinella G. Laparoscopic sacrocolpopexy in the treatment of vaginal vault prolapse: 8 years experience. Eur J Obstet Gynecol Reprod Biol. 2009;146(2):227–31.
12. Sergent F, Resch B, Loisel C, Bisson V, Schaal JP, Marpeau L. Mid-term outcome of laparoscopic sacrocolpopexy with anterior and posterior polyester mesh for the treatment of genitourinary prolapse. Eur J Obstet Gynecol Reprod Biol. 2011;156:217–22.
13. Sarlos D, Kots L, Ryu G, Schaer G. Long-term follow-up of laparoscopic sacrocolpopexy. Int Urogynecol J. 2014;25(9):1207–12.
14. Bui C, Ballester M, Chereau E, Guillo E, Darai E. Functional results and quality of life of laparoscopic promontofixation in the cure of genital prolapse. Gynecol Obstet Fertil. 2010;38:563–8.
15. Rivoire C, Botchorishvili R, Canis M, Jardon K, Rabischong B, Wattiez A, Mage G. Complete laparoscopic treatment of genital prolapse with meshes including vaginal promontofixation and anterior repair: a series of 138 patients. J Minim Invasive Gynecol. 2007;14(6):712–8.
16. Marcus-Braun N, von Theobald P. Mesh removal following transvaginal mesh placement: a case series of 104 operations. Int Urogynecol J. 2010;21(4):423–30.
17. Fischer JP, Basta MN, Mirzabeigi MN, Bauder AR, Fox JP, Drebin JA, Serletti JM, Kovach SJ. A risk model and cost analysis of incisional hernia after elective, abdominal surgery based upon 12,373 cases: the case for targeted prophylactic intervention. Ann Surg. 2015;28. [Epub ahead of print]
18. Kdous M, Zhioua F. 3-year results of transvaginal cystocele repair with transobturator four-arm mesh: a prospective study of 105 patients. Arab J Urol. 2014;12(4):275–84.
19. de Tayrac R, Brouziyne M, Priou G, Devoldère G, Marie G, Renaudie J. Transvaginal repair of stage III-IV cystocele using a lightweight mesh: safety and 36-month outcome. Int Urogynecol J. 2015;26(8):1147–54.
20. Lucot JP, Fritel X, Debodinance P, Bader G, Cosson M, Giraudet G, Collinet P, Rubod C, Fernandez H, Fournet S, Lesavre M, Deffieux X, Faivre E, Trichot C, Demoulin G, Jacquetin B, Savary D, Botchorichvili R, Campagne Loiseau S, Salet-Lizee D, Villet R, Gadonneix P, Delporte P, Ferry P, Aucouturier JS, Thirouard Y, de Tayrac R, Fatton B, Wagner L, Nadeau C, Wattiez A, Garbin O, Youssef Azer Akladios C, Thoma V, Baulon Thaveau E, Saussine C, Hermieu JF, Delmas V, Blanc S, Tardif D, Fauconnier A, GROG (groupe de recherche en gynécologie et obstétrique). PROSPERE randomized controlled trial: laparoscopic sacropexy versus vaginal mesh for cystocele POP repair. J Gynecol Obstet Biol Reprod. 2013;42(4):334–41.
21. David V, Géraldine G, Jean-Philippe L, Hélène B, Michel C. Impact of laparoscopic sacrocolpopexy learning curve on operative time, perioperative complications and short term results. Eur J Obstet Gynecol Reprod Biol. 2015;191:84–9.

How to Select Patients to Improve Results?

Patient selection is a direct consequence of the long term results study. Once again, the goal is to master enough different techniques to be able to select the best procedure for each patient. But patient selection depends also on your level of skill. In your early experience, choose easy patients to start and validate your learning curve.

1. What is an "easy" patient? The main features that can make your operation difficult, are:

    (a) Previous pelvic or abdominal operations generating adhesions. Operations addressing deep endometriosis, adnexal abscesses, peritonitis of any origin, myomectomies, bowel resections, are likely to induce heavy adhesions. It is almost always possible to free the pelvis laparoscopically, but the risk of bowel or bladder injury is much higher. It is sometimes difficult to find the way of the ureters. Please note that previous Cesarean section can be an issue; it may make the bladder dissection more difficult and increases the risk of injury.

    (b) Obesity. Fatty tissue infiltrates the peritoneum and makes it difficult to localize and to dissect the promontory. The pararectal fossa is also infiltrated and this tissue is richly vascularized. Blunt dissection may provoke much more bleeding than in normal weighted patients. The mesosigmoid and the mesentery is very thick and heavy and vascularized, making it difficult to push away the bowel. The procedure will require a higher CO_2 pressure (up to 15 mm Hg) and a stronger Trendelenbourg position and your anesthesiologist will be in trouble. Very frequently, obese patients have colic diverticulitis which makes the sigmoid rigid, inflammatory and fragile. If I certainly never would recommend to start your learning curve with obese patients, it is obvious that these women have the best indication for LSCP: laparoscopy is minimal invasive, mesh surgery is always required in these patients who have a very high risk of recurrence and many are diabetic with a high risk of infection after vaginal insertion of the mesh.

© Springer International Publishing AG 2017   81
P. von Theobald, *Laparoscopic Sacrocolpopexy for Beginners*,
DOI 10.1007/978-3-319-57636-7_10

(c) Vault prolapse. This is a very good indication for LSCP but the dissection of the vault is not always easy. Usually, the bladder bends over the vaginal scar of the previous hysterectomy and sticks to it. You will have to free completely the vaginal cuff in order to apply the mesh of de-peritonized tissue in order to facilitate tissue incorporation. Posterior dissection is usually easy and quick because the distance to the levator ani muscles is short. Further, if the hysterectomy has been performed with a laparotomy, you may have to face adhesions as well. Last point: if the cervix or the uterus is present, it is easy to fix the meshes to the cervix or the isthmus. The fixation is very strong. At the opposite, if there's no solid structure, you'll have to fix the meshes to the vaginal fascia that is usually this and weak. You'll have to be careful to avoid transfixing sutures through the vaginal wall. And you will have to apply a big number of sutures to avoid the tearing away of the vault from the mesh at first coughing when the patient wakes up.

To summarize: an easy patient is a woman of normal weight who has no previous history of surgery likely to provoke adhesions and who still has her uterus.

2. Patient selection according to the POP:
   (a) Good indications:
   - Level 1 defect: enterocele, uterine descent (hysterocele) without cervical elongation. The perfect indication if isolated.
   - Level 2 posterior defect: rectocele, especially if associated with level 1 defect.
   - Recurrence after vaginal repair. Failures of sacrospinous fixation or high Mc Call procedure are excellent indications. Recurrence after vaginal repair with mesh is a good indication as well; frequently, it is possible to find the vaginal inserted meshes ad suture le laparoscopic mesh to them.
   - POP with pelvic pain. POP is never painful; only pelvic heaviness may be related to POP. If there is pelvic pain and if this pain cannot be explained by clinical investigation and radiology, the laparoscopic approach may be useful to find an etiology at the time of the prolapse repair. Endometriosis, Masters and Allen's syndrome, diverticulitis, adhesions may be found.
   (b) Bad indications:
   - Big cystocele with lateral defect. The recurrence rate is above 50% and, as the recurrence occurs rather quickly, it frequently looks more like an incomplete treatment than like a recurrence. Big cystoceles include most frequently a lateral defect, possibly associated to other defects. Big cystoceles are rare in POP in the young women before 50. After menopausal, cystocele is very often associated to any POP.
   - Recurrence after previous SCP or LSCP. In this case, the POP doesn't usually involve level 1 and a vaginal repair with or without mesh is the easiest approach. Frequently, you'll find the SCP mesh during dissection and you'll be able to fix the vaginal mesh or the fascial repair to this LCP mesh. Recurrence after SCP is most frequently a cystocele (as demonstrated in our

series) or an elongation of the cervix (trachelocele) that you just have to shorten to bring the cervix back to a normal length.

- If level 1 is involved in the recurrence, it seems logical to try a vaginal sacrospinous fixation (SSF) because the dissection stays retroperitoneal and is not affected by peritoneal adhesion or fibrosis around the SCP mesh. We use to perform it bilaterally with a dedicated device like the Mya Hook (re usable) or the Capio (Boston Scientific) or the Digitex (Coloplast). We have performed more than ten of these procedures after SCP failure without major difficulty and with very good results.

- But LSCP is possible after failed SCP. We have performed six of these operations after failed SCP and then failed SSF. You have to cut the mesh coming from the promontory and let it attached to it. It will be useful to suspend the new meshes without having to dissect again the promontory. Vaginal dissection, of course, is very tough and risky in these patients. Furthermore, the left ureter is always very close to the mesh, attracted by the fibrosis generated by the implant. Not to recommend for beginners!

To conclude, your first ten patients should be skinny, have no previous history of heavy pelvic surgery or total hysterectomy, present a level 1 defect (uterine descent and accompanying enterocele, maybe have a rectocele but no major cystocele and no lateral defect at clinical examination. After the 10 first patients, you can start to include vault prolapse and after 30 patients extend to moderately obese patients.

Post Operative Care

11

1. During hospital stay: Hospital stay is usually no more than 24 h. We have performed LSCP on a few out patients; it is possible to do so but most of women prefer staying one night at hospital in our population. Foley catheter can be removed after 6 h and the patient can eat and rise. At this stage, you have to check for complications like bowel occlusion, abdominal wall hematoma, infection and urinary retention, especially if a sub urethral sling has been inserted. The woman can be discharged as soon as everything is back to normal function.
2. After discharge, post operative care relies on precise and complete counseling of the patient. These are the main items to be discussed with the patient.
   (a) No sports during one month. After that period, avoid sports like running, jumping (tennis, Zumba …), horse riding, during one more month. Prefer swimming, stretching, walking, aso..). Two months after LSCP, the meshes are supposed to be totally incorporated into live connective tissue and activity may go back to normal without restriction.
   (b) Sexual activity: No intercourse during one month is the rule.
   (c) Professional activity: The patient may resume professional activity rather quickly after one week depending on the type of activity. If it involves carrying heavy weights (>5 kg), or if it requires physical strength (cleaning rooms, gardening …), return to normal activity should be delayed after one month.
   (d) Constipation may be pre existing to LSCP. In this case, a treatment should be found before the procedure and carried out at least during 6 months after. In 20–30% of patients, LSCP induces constipation in the early post operative course. It may be due to the pre sacral dissection that may irritate or injury the pre sacral nervous plexus and provoke a kind of rectoplegia. Post LSCP constipation may last during 3–6 months before resolution in most patients. It is crucial to treat constipation and obstructed defecation in the post operative months because hard pushing may distend or break the mesh fixations. It is a risk factor for POP and also for recurrence, of course. I use to tell my

© Springer International Publishing AG 2017
P. von Theobald, *Laparoscopic Sacrocolpopexy for Beginners*,
DOI 10.1007/978-3-319-57636-7_11

patients when they leave the hospital, to take systematically some oral laxatives during 3 months and to adapt the doses in order to have an easy defecation.

(e) The one month follow up is very important to check wound healing, to establish a POP Q score, to examine the vagina to make sure that there's no transfixiating suture visible. This consultation will reinsure the patient before returning to normal life. It's necessary to tell the patient that LSCP has corrected the anatomy but that normal function of the concerned organs will take 3–6 months to recover. Moderate pelvic pain, due to the dissection, to the sutures or, very frequently, to the trocar incisions, may be present. It will resolve spontaneously but can be improved with soft analgesic drugs. If bowel problems exist, like difficult defecation, they should be managed very seriously. Obstructed micturition is rare at this stage but urgency and frequency are frequently reported and may require prescription of anti-cholinergic drugs during one or two months. Urinary Stress Incontinence (USI) may appear just after LSCP as after any POP repair. Usually, the patient is aware of it if you did good preoperative information. One month after the operation, it's too early to indicate a sling operation which can be discussed after 3–6 months if it persists. I ask the patient to try some pelvic floor rehabilitation and check again after 2 months.

If a prolapse is present at 1 month, it can be because of an early recurrence due to constipation or heavy coughing after LSCP or, most frequently, to insufficient surgical correction, mainly in case of cystocele with lateral defect.

If the patient is satisfied and everything well, a control at 1 year is strongly recommended even if you're not intending to publish a series. If there's a problem, a monthly control should be programmed until the patient is fine.

Alternative Techniques: Which and When?

12

Describing alternative techniques and their indications would require a whole book. The aim of this section is to orientate the young surgeon to find a way out when LSCP is not possible or failed. We will very shortly describe the techniques and give a reference in literature for further information. We will also underline the situations in which the alternative technique could be used.

1. Alternative procedures for level 1 defect:
   (a) Laparoscopic fixation to the uterosacral ligaments [1, 2]. Instead of using meshes, you can use the uterosacral ligaments to suspend the vaginal wall or the cervix or shorten the uterosacral ligaments with sutures. This may be associated to a Douglassectomy or a culdoplasty. There are only few reports of results in literature and no serious comparison to other techniques. In fact, if the uterosacral ligaments are of poor quality, this procedure is not feasible. In some POP patients, the uterosacral ligaments are even not visible because of distension or atrophy. This technique should be considered when a rectal injury occurs during posterior dissection, contra indicating the use of a synthetic mesh.
   (b) Laparoscopic fixation to the pelvic sidewall [3]. This is the technique promoted since years by my old friend Jean Bernard Dubuisson from Geneva. It is based on an old open procedure that had been abandoned because of the high rate of enterocele occurring after this operation due to the axis of tension that opens the Douglas pouch. JB Dubuisson wanted to find a procedure that could avoid the dissection of the promontory and of the recto vaginal plane. A pre cut mesh is introduced through a lateral skin incision and pushed through the extra peritoneal space under laparoscopic view control from one side to the other and sutured to the vault or the isthmus. In order to prevent the high risk of enterocele, a culdoplasty has to be performed in order to close the Douglas pouch. This technique could be useful when the promontory is not accessible.

© Springer International Publishing AG 2017
P. von Theobald, *Laparoscopic Sacrocolpopexy for Beginners*,
DOI 10.1007/978-3-319-57636-7_12

(c) Anterior hysteropexy (ventrofixation) [4, 5]. This is a very old operation (but easy and quick to perform) has been described since the nineteenth century and published in 1915 [4]. It has been abandoned because the fixation of the uterus to the abdominal wall modifies the vaginal axis and opens widely the Douglas pouch. Consecutive enterocele is almost systematic inducing pain and defecation problems as seen in unintentional uterine ventrofixation due to repeated caesarian section. Some authors [5] have suggested that a poor open operation could be a good laparoscopic operation mainly because it's easy to perform. That's not our way of thinking. We don't recommend uterine ventrofixation in any situation.

(d) Vaginal sacrospinous ligament fixation [1, 6, 7]. Initially described by Richter, this fixation of the vaginal vault to the sacrospinous ligament is usually done unilaterally and with sutures. Many variations exist. It can be performed bilaterally. It can be reinforced by a mesh. It can be done under direct view of the ligament presented with three retractors or under "fingertip control", blindly with the help of a device. Many devices, reusable (Miya Hook, SeraPro) or not (Digitex, Capio), are on the market. Results are very satisfying. A recent meta analysis [1] seems to indicate that sacrospinous ligament fixation is slightly less effective than SCP on the results but sacrospinous ligament fixation has less complications and a lower cost. It remains an excellent technique for level 1 defect and we recommend this technique in vault prolapse as a first line. It is also very useful in level 1 recurrence after LSCP because the dissection remains extra peritoneal, avoiding the abdominal adhesions around the mesh. Frequently, vaginal dissection may lead you to find the abdominal mesh and you can suture it to the vaginal vault or the uterine cervix instead of fixing to the sacrospinous ligament.

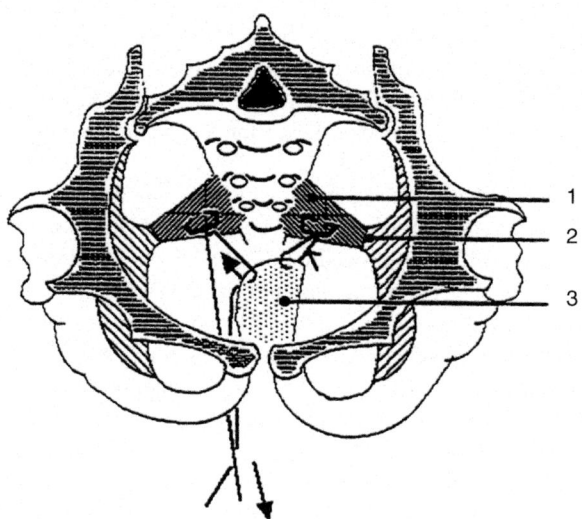

Figure: Bilateral sacrospinous ligament fixation (*1* sacrospinous ligament, *2* ischial spine, *3* vaginal vault)

(e) Vaginal fixation to the uterosacral ligaments [8–10]. Again an old but efficient technique. Vaginal uterosacral ligament suspension seems to be as effective as vaginal [8]. The main risk is the proximity of the ureters that may lead to ligature or kinking. The poor quality of the uterosacral ligaments in many POP patients may also impair the long term results. We prefer to do a sacrospinous ligament fixation for all these reasons.

(f) Lefort's procedure (or other vaginal closure technique) [11–13]. This is a very effective operation for patients above 70 or 80 years old having no more desire for vaginal intercourse. Colpocleisis can be performed safely without vaginal hysterectomy, on a day surgery and under local anesthesia. The technique (photos below) is very elegant with an effectiveness of almost 100% and very few side effects.

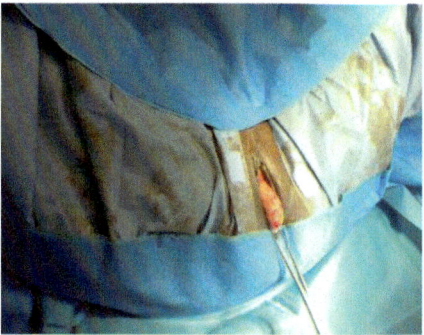

Total prolapse

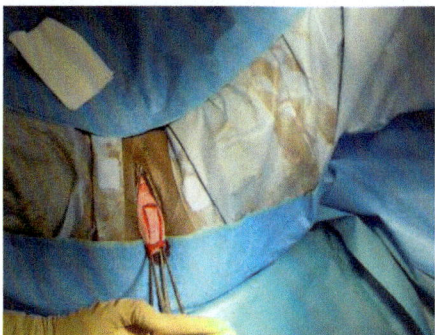

Step 1: Anterior incision

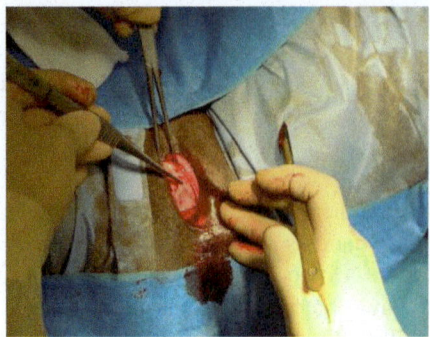

Step 2: Posterior incision

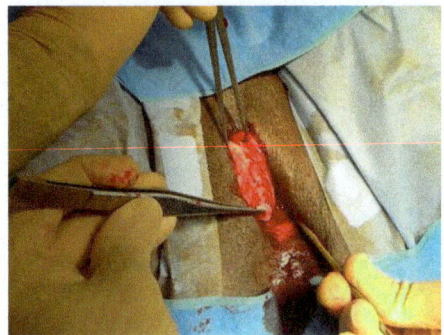

Step 3: Remove mucosa

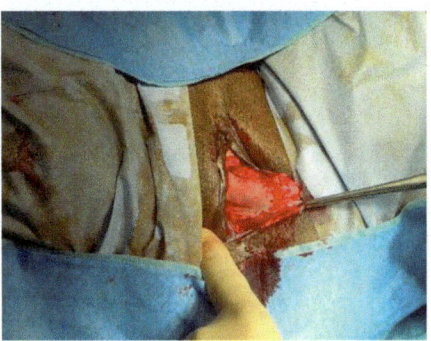

Remaining mucosa on the right

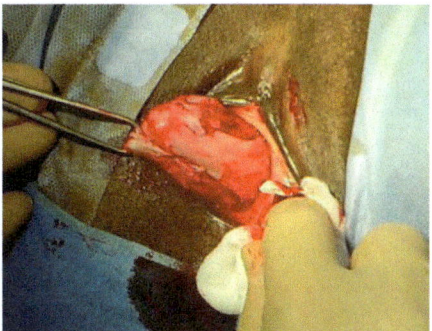

Remaining mucosa on the left

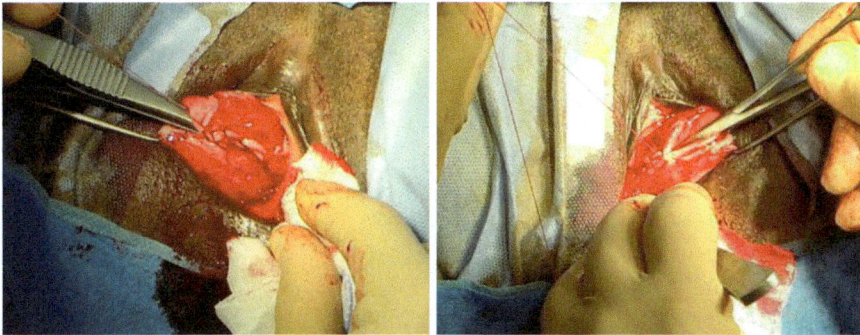

Step 4: Continuous sutures to build right and left tunnel

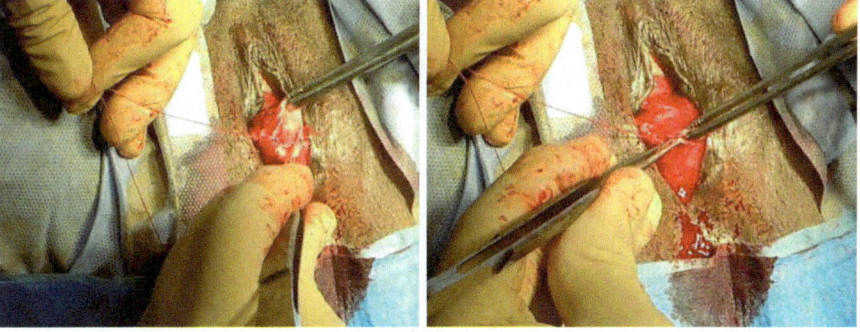

Step 5: The mucosa is closed in front of the cervix

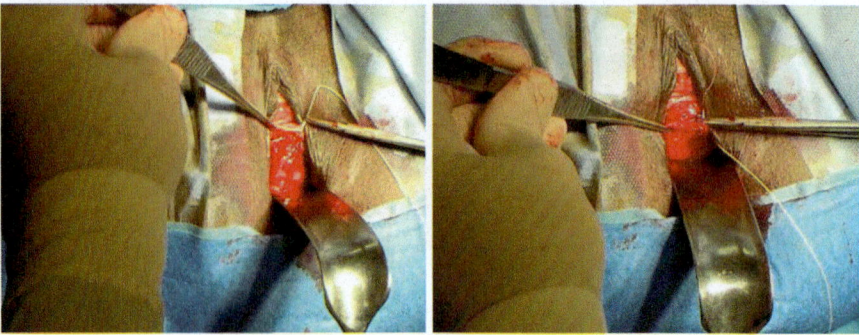

Step 6: Closure of the vagina

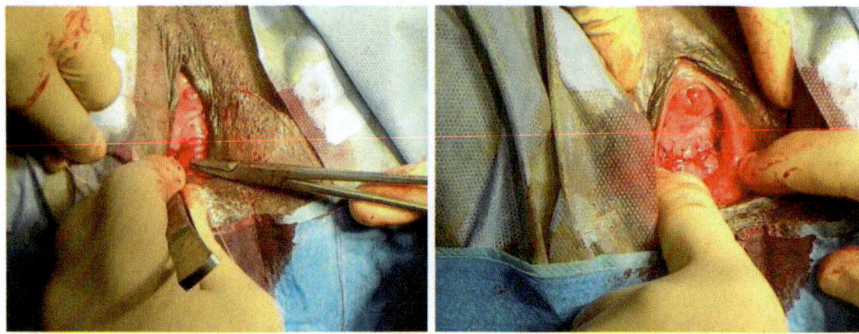

Step 6: Closure of the vagina

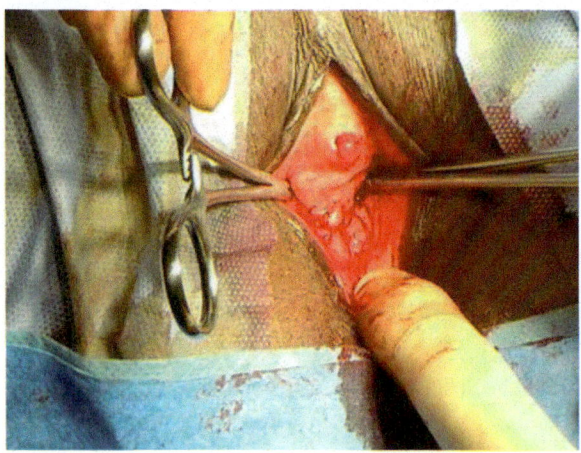

Final view with the two lateral tunnels

2. Alternative procedures for level 2 posterior defect:

   (a) Laparoscopic rectopexy [14] is indicated in case of obstructed defecation due to rectal intussusceptions (see picture below), associated or not to a rectocele or a total rectal prolapse. More than an alternative technique, laparoscopic rectopexy can be an additional step to LSCP after a multidisciplinary approach of heavy defecation dysfunction. The technique and the dissection are very similar to LSCP (see picture below).

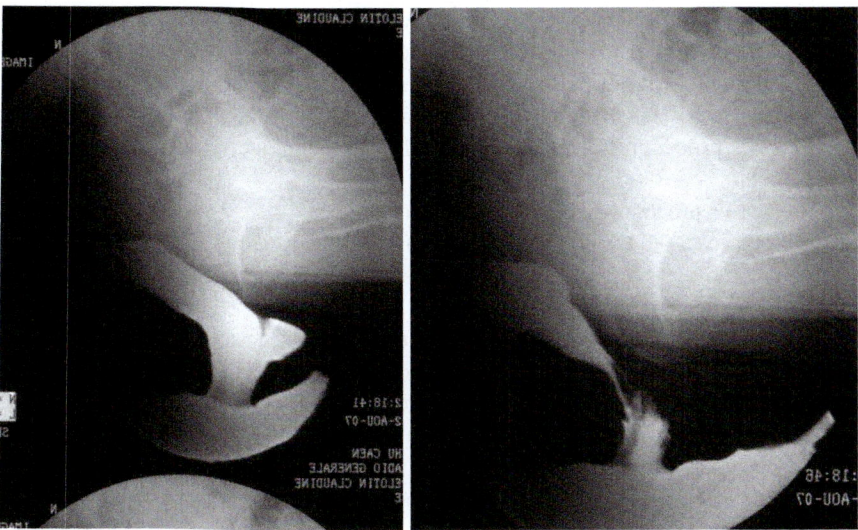

Picture: Rectal intussusception at defecography

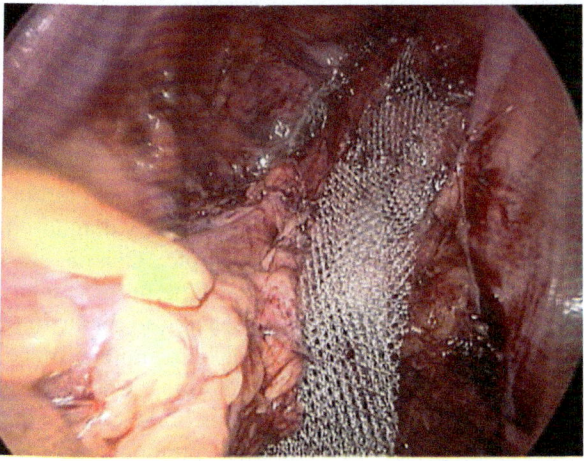

Picture: Laparoscopic rectopexy according to Orr Loygue

(b) Vaginal fascia autologous tissue repair. Here's not the place for that old and big debate about autologous or synthetic mesh repair. The main procedures used to repair posterior level 2 defect are fascia repair, vaginal skin bridge techniques and levator ani myorraphy. Vaginal posterior colpectomy is only the excision of redundant distended vaginal skin but not a way to repair the rectocele. Recurrence rate after posterior autologous tissue level 2 repairs is much lower than in the anterior compartment and recurrence occurs much later. Current recommendations for vaginal POP surgery go for this kind of repair.

(c) Vaginal posterior mesh repair [15] keeps a place in case of recurrence after vaginal autologous tissue repair or after LSCP. Frequently, you may find the abdominal mesh during the dissection and you can suture the vaginal mesh to the previously laparoscopically inserted mesh to cover the defect.

(d) Lefort's procedure (or other vaginal closure technique) works also in level 2 defects.

3. Alternative procedures for level 2 anterior defect:

(a) Laparoscopic Burch procedure or para vaginal repair [16]. These procedures are aiming to reinsert the structures on their lateral attachments, according to Richardson. Burch colposuspension, that had some effect on stress incontinence, was at the origin supposed to cure also cystocele. It was not very efficient and, in the same way, laparoscopic paravaginal repair doesn't seem to be associated with very good outcomes in literature. This may be due to the fact that the anatomy of the Retzius space remains confidential among surgeons. Structures are not so easy to identify. Cure rates vary between 60 and 80%. Our suggestion in case of lateral defect is to perform a vaginal repair with mesh.

(b) Vaginal autologous tissue repair. The debate is still running. Modern anatomists like DeLancey [17] and Petros [18] have perfectly identified the possible defects. Rupture or distension may be medial like a hernia through the fascia, sometimes focal, sometimes extensive. The injury may be lateral, detaching the vaginal fascia from the pelvic sidewall. It may also be an upper defect, if the fascia is detached from the pericervical ring. The consequence of this advanced anatomical knowledge was the birth of the "site specific surgery of POP". The aim was to avoid a global repair, already known as painful and causing vagina narrowing. The site-specific procedure intended to reattach the disrupted fascia or ligament in its correct position, once the defect was perfectly diagnosed. The problem is that in most patients, defects are multiple. Thus, a site-specific repair becomes frequently more or less global. The more you have to pull on a weak, thin and distorted fascia, using tension to repair it, the more it will get thinner, weaker and likely to break in another place. Tension full suture is always fragile and painful. Nothing was done to improve the quality of the tissue. One of the principles of the classical techniques is to treat the colpoceles by excising the redundant vaginal wall tissue. Colpectomy was one of the main components of the repair procedures, aiming to narrow the vagina to its "normal size"! Probably because the vagina is a virtual cavity, the colpectomies were frequently very extensive. The colporraphies, myorraphies and perineorraphies were very tight, in order to let nothing come out of the vulva. Frequently also, these tight repairs were causing pain and dyspareunia. The problem is that none of these traditional techniques are the same. Colpotomies are different: horizontal, vertical, T-shaped, Y-shaped, diamond shaped … Fascia dissections are very various: complete dissection, dissection from the vaginal wall, dissection from the bladder or rectum, no dissection …. Repairs are widely various: simple suture, overlapping suture, purse suture, multiple transversal sutures …. To summarize, we can say that the traditional repair is not standardized and that it is aiming through very various means to repair defects by stretching and reattaching autologous tissue, to narrow the vagina and vulva to prevent a descent of any kind. Recurrence rate for cystocele is between 30 and 50% after a follow up of 2 years in literature. We don't recommend it except for patients with high risk of infection like immune depressed or unstable diabetics.

(c) Vaginal mesh repair [19]: Three main principles are leading to a successful repair with meshes: **the bio surgery of the collagen** (or directed healing process), the **correction of the anatomical axes** of the vagina and **the tissue sparing approach**.

Bio surgery of the collagen: this concept has been invented by Hubert Manhès in the early 90s, when he intended to correct cystocoele by laparoscopy with a mesh in the Retzius space held only by fibrin glue and a pessary. In fact, when you insert a mesh in any tissue, it will involve a foreign body reaction. Fibrin due to the dissection will quickly surround the mesh, giving a soft primary hold. Granulocytes and macrophages will colonise the mesh within 48 h in the process of the inflammatory response. After a week, fibroblasts will appear on the mesh, starting to produce the extra cellular matrix of a new connective tissue around the mesh. Thus, the goal of the mesh is mainly to "stake" the building of this fresh new connective tissue in the correct dissection plane, in the right direction. This tissue, being continuous with the pelvic fascias and ligaments around it, will be more resistant to tearing and traction than any suture could be by itself. The tissue in growth of the mesh is the key of resistance, not the mesh itself. Since connective tissue is a live tissue, it needs to be continuously remodelled to stay resistant and elastic, the proteic matrix needs to be renewed. Especially in these POP patients, whose collagen is of poor quality (if it was strong, they would not have developed a POP). If an absorbable mesh is inserted, it will induce an inflammatory response followed by macrophages, fibroblasts and a new fascia or ligament will be produced on this site. But when the mesh is finally absorbed, the new collagen will age and undergo the natural evolution of the autologous one, which is poor. If a non absorbable mesh is used, the foreign body reaction will persist and the collagen will be renewed on a regular basis around the mesh and the quality of the new ligament or fascia will stay constant. Another very important feature of the prostheses has to be underlined here: the pore size. Implantation of a polypropylene thread provokes a foreign body reaction with fibrosis around it. If two threads are too close, the fibrosis will be continuous, involving rigidity and retraction. The complication rate is reduced with larger pores. As the result of the repair is not due to the resistance of the mesh itself, but to the neofibrogenesis involved, large pore sizes must be used.

The correction of the anatomical axes of the vagina: The vagina is a very sophisticated anatomical structure (figure below) and its perfect reconstruction is a real challenge. But the results of pelvic floor surgery depend on this anatomical correction. The vagina starts at the vulva as a vertical slot, crosses the elevator plate aiming towards L5–S1 and then the posterior vaginal wall lies on the elevator plate, aiming towards S3. The vagina is ending as a horizontal slot. Thus, increasing intraabdominal pressure at effort will apply the horizontally flat upper third of the vagina on the elevator plate (if it is in the right place, maintained by the utero sacral and cardinal ligaments). Meanwhile, the puborectalis will increase the angulation between upper and lower third of the vagina, compressing laterally the vagina and closing the vertical slot portion. This functional anatomy is related to balanced forces as described by Peter Petros in his Integral Theory. Pelvic floor repair should aim to restore these forces without any over tensioning. Overcorrection of one segment will always lead to pain, dysfunction or breaking involved by increased tension on another segment.

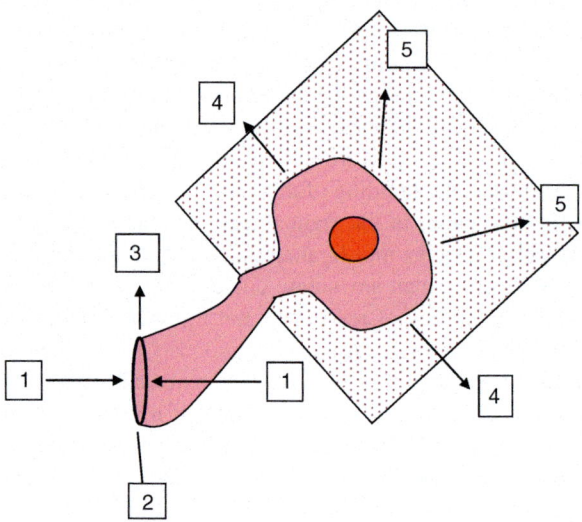

Figure: Three dimensional view of the vagina (*1* bulbocavernous muscles, *2* perineal body, *3* pubourethral ligament, *4* cardinal ligaments, *5* uterosacral ligaments)

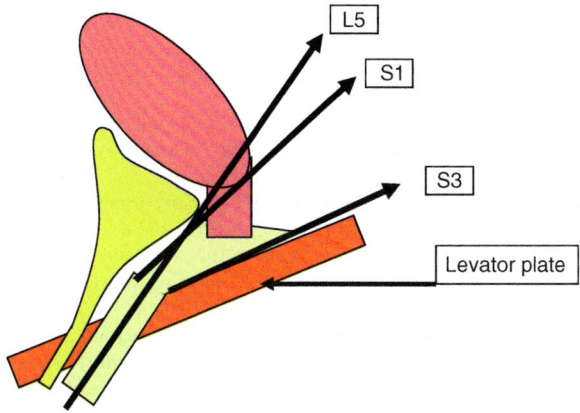

Figure: Axes of the vagina

The tissue sparing approach: Colpectomy aims to trim the excessive vaginal epithelium in order to "tailor" a "normal looking" vagina. But vaginal epithelium is a live tissue, it is able to recover after incision and distension. For instance, after distension by vaginal delivery, it retracts back to its normal size after a couple of hours. After abdominal or laparoscopic sacrocolpopexy (almost never associated with a colpectomy), it retracts to a normal shape within a few days. Of course, at the end of the surgery, a trimmed vaginal wall looks better because it is not redundant. But, as soon as the patient rises from bed or when the bladder or the rectum fills, it is under tension and its thickness is reduced as is its vascularisation and innervation. This is crucial if you use meshes to reinforce the fascia; a local necrosis of the over-lying epithelium will expose the prosthesis and result in erosion. It may also be a problem in conventional surgery and explain some of the frequent recurrences mainly in cystoceles; sometimes the vaginal mucosa is so thin that you almost can see the bladder through it. The main difference between traditional vaginal POP surgery and mesh surgery is that the first is treating anterior and posterior colpoceles and the latter is treating cystoceles and rectoceles.

Who should benefit from vaginal anterior mesh surgery? All patients with a symptomatic large sized cystocele, especially if there's a lateral defect (79). The aim is here to have a perfectly standardized technique, an easy learning curve and to offer every patient a painless, minimal invasive, long term effective operation.

References

1. Barber MD, Maher C. Apical prolapse. Int Urogynecol J. 2013 Nov;24(11):1815–33.
2. Filmar GA, Fisher HW, Aranda E, Lotze PM. Laparoscopic uterosacral ligament suspension and sacral colpopexy: results and complications. Int Urogynecol J. 2014 Dec;25(12):1645–53.
3. Dubuisson J, Veit-Rubin N, Bouquet de Jolinière J, Dubuisson JB. Laparoscopic lateral suspension: benefits of a cross-shaped mesh to treat difficult vaginal vault prolapse. J Minim Invasive Gynecol. 2016 Jul–Aug;23(5):672.

4. O'Conor J. A mode for ventrofixation of the uterus for the relief of prolapsus. Ann Surg. 1915 Oct;62(4):479–80.
5. Shalev E, Bustan M, Peleg D. Laparoscopic Ventrofixation: an alternate treatment approach for uterine prolapse. J Gynecol Surg. 1996;12(2):105–7.
6. Friedman T, Neuman M, Peled Y, Krissi H. A new reusable suturing device for vaginal sacro-spinous fixation: feasibility and safety study. Eur J Obstet Gynecol Reprod Biol. 2015 Oct;193:23–6.
7. Vaudano G, Gatti M. Correction of vaginal vault prolapse using Capio™ suture capturing device: our experience. Minerva Ginecol. 2015 Apr;67(2):103–11.
8. Turner LC, Lavelle ES, Shepherd JP. Comparison of complications and prolapse recurrence between laparoscopic and vaginal uterosacral ligament suspension for the treatment of vaginal prolapse. Int Urogynecol J. 2016 May;27(5):797–803.
9. Spelzini F, Frigerio M, Manodoro S, Interdonato ML, Cesana MC, Verri D, Fumagalli C, Sicuri M, Nicoli E, Polizzi S, Milani R. Modified McCall culdoplasty versus Shull suspension in pelvic prolapse primary repair: a retrospective study. Int Urogynecol J. 2016 Apr;5. [Epub ahead of print]
10. Milani R, Frigerio M, Manodoro S, Cola A, Spelzini F. Transvaginal uterosacral ligament hysteropexy: a retrospective feasibility study. Int Urogynecol J. 2016 May;19. [Epub ahead of print]
11. Ng SC, Chen GD. Obliterative LeFort colpocleisis for pelvic organ prolapse in elderly women aged 70 years and over. Taiwan J Obstet Gynecol. 2016 Feb;55(1):68–71.
12. Linder BJ, Gebhart JB, Occhino JA. Total colpocleisis: technical considerations. Int Urogynecol J. 2016 May;14. [Epub ahead of print]
13. Jones KA, Zhuo Y, Solak S, Harmanli O. Hysterectomy at the time of colpocleisis: a decision analysis. Int Urogynecol J. 2016 May;27(5):805–10.
14. Horisberger K, Rickert A, Templin S, Post S, Kienle P. Laparoscopic ventral mesh rectopexy in complex pelvic floor disorder. Int J Color Dis. 2016 May;31(5):991–6.
15. von Theobald P. Place of mesh in vaginal surgery, including its removal and revision. Best Pract Res Clin Obstet Gynaecol. 2011 Apr;25(2):197–203.
16. Hosni MM, El-Feky AE, Agur WI, Khater EM. Evaluation of three different surgical approaches in repairing paravaginal support defects: a comparative trial. Arch Gynecol Obstet. 2013 Dec;288(6):1341–8.
17. Stein TA, DeLancey JO. Structure of the perineal membrane in females: gross and microscopic anatomy. Obstet Gynecol. 2008;111(3):686–93.
18. Petros PE, Ulmsten UI. An integral theory and its method for the diagnosis and management of female urinary incontinence. Scand J Urol Nephrol Suppl. 1993;153:1–93.
19. Von Theobald P, Zimmermann CW, Davila GW. New techniques in genital prolapse surgery. London: Springer; 2011.

Conclusion of the Author

13

After 35 years of intensive professional life in the field of surgical gynecology and urogynecology, I feel very happy to have had the opportunity to live in a fascinating period of very quick evolution. In 1985, when we performed our first laparoscopic salpingectomy for an ectopic pregnancy, my old professor and mentor called us irresponsible, almost criminal. Two years later, in 1987, when I started as a consultant in his department, he called me to his office and told me to buy a video camera and to develop laparoscopic surgery that he thought to be the future. At that moment, everything was new and open, the instruments had to be designed, the techniques to be adapted from laparotomy. Laparoscopic surgery spread very quickly in France and Germany. We wanted to prove that every operation could be performed laparoscopically. And, of course, we went too far. Open surgery and vaginal surgery are in fact not competing techniques but complementary procedures with specific indications. Concerning POP repair, in the eighties, open SCP and vaginal techniques like colporrhaphy, fascial repair, sacrospinous ligament fixation were the rule. Open surgeons claimed their technique (born in the 50s) was the gold standard certainly thought that the main reason for vaginal surgery was that the surgeon was not able to perform SCP. Vaginal claimed their technique was less dangerous, site specific and not less efficient. In 1992–1993, three French gynecologists performed the first LSCP in order to combine the efficiency of mesh insertion, reinforcing the weak, distended native tissue, to the minimal invasiveness of laparoscopy. The idea was great and series started to be published in 2000–2001 with good results, similar to those of open approach. But the learning curve was rather long and LSCP didn't spread very quickly and the long term results on anterior defect were not as good as expected. Furthermore, at the same time, at the end of the 90s, vaginal surgery moved quickly forwards with the beginning of vaginal mesh insertion. That was supposed to be the revenge of the "poor" vaginal surgeons. The combination of the effectiveness of native tissue reinforcement with mesh as in LSCP with the minimal invasiveness and the short learning curve of vaginal POP surgery. No more need to spent time on learning tough laparoscopic techniques. Here again, we went too quickly too far. Inappropriate and sometimes dangerous materials were

© Springer International Publishing AG 2017
P. von Theobald, *Laparoscopic Sacrocolpopexy for Beginners*,
DOI 10.1007/978-3-319-57636-7_13

commercialized. The learning curve of vaginal POP surgery especially with implants was largely underestimated. In 2010, the FDA gave a warning about vaginal mesh surgery and a lot of American companies left the market. Some surgeons went back to traditional vaginal surgery, back to the nineteenth century techniques. But many others knew that a mesh technique is needed in POP surgery, even if it isn't for every patient. Most of urogynecologic surgeons know now that one technique cannot solve every clinical situation. Like always, evolution goes like a pendulum; it goes one direction but always too far. Then it goes back and there too, always too far. Vaginal and laparoscopic POP surgery have gone that way and I hope it will stabilize some day. "In medium stat virtus", like always. My credo has always been to train as much as needed to be able to perform any surgery, vaginal and laparoscopic, and to indicate the approach according to the patient's clinical status. Since the mid 90s, I perform 70% vaginal and 30% laparoscopic surgery for POP. And vaginal mesh surgery seems to have a strong indication, more and more proven by EBM, mainly for large cystoceles. LSCP is one of my favorite operations. It's a very anatomical, bloodless dissection. Results are rather good, even 20 years later if the indication is correct. The learning curve is long but it's worth investing time in a technique you can't get away from if you want to be a modern urogynecologic surgeon.

Index

© Springer International Publishing AG 2017
P. von Theobald, *Laparoscopic Sacrocolpopexy for Beginners*,
DOI 10.1007/978-3-319-57636-7

The manufacturer's authorised representative in the EU is Springer
Nature Customer Service Centre GmbH, Europaplatz 3, 69115 Heidelberg,
Germany. If you have any concerns regarding our products, please
contact ProductSafety@springernature.com

Printed and bound by CPI Group (UK) Ltd, Croydon, CR0 4YY
23/04/2026
02095596-0003